NATURAL HEALING HANDBOOK

Body Movement
for inner harmony

NATURAL HEALING HANDBOOK

Body Movement
for inner harmony

TUCKER • EVANS • HUDSON • MACDONNELL

LORENZ BOOKS

This edition is published by Lorenz Books

Lorenz Books is an imprint of Anness Publishing Ltd
Hermes House, 88–89 Blackfriars Road, London SE1 8HA
tel. 020 7401 2077; fax 020 7633 9499
www.lorenzbooks.com; info@anness.com

© Anness Publishing Ltd 2001, 2002
Published in the USA by Lorenz Books, Anness Publishing Inc., 27 West 20th Street, New York, NY 10011;
fax 212 807 6813

This edition distributed in the UK by Aurum Press Ltd, 25 Bedford Avenue, London WC1B 3AT;
tel. 020 7637 3225; fax 020 7580 2469

This edition distributed in the USA by National Book Network, 4720 Boston Way, Lanham, MD 20706;
tel. 301 459 3366; fax 301 459 1705; www.nbnbooks.com

This edition distributed in Canada by General Publishing, 895 Don Mills Road, 400–402 Park Centre, Toronto,
Ontario M3C 1W3; tel. 416 445 3333; fax 416 445 5991; www.genpub.com

This edition distributed in Australia by Pan Macmillan Australia, Level 18, St Martins Tower, 31 Market St,
Sydney, NSW 2000; tel. 1300 135 113; fax 1300 135 103; email customer.service@macmillan.com.au

This edition distributed in New Zealand by David Bateman Ltd, 30 Tarndale Grove, Off Bush Road, Albany,
Auckland; tel. (09) 415 7664; fax (09) 415 8892

All rights reserved. No part of this publication may be reproduced, stored in a retrieval system, or transmitted
in any way or by any means, electronic, mechanical, photocopying, recording or otherwise, without the prior
written permission of the copyright holder.

A CIP catalogue record for this book is available from the British Library.

Publisher: Joanna Lorenz
Managing Editor: Helen Sudell
Project Editor: Emma Gray
Designer: Balley Design Associates
Main photographers: Don Last and Dave Jordan
Production Controller: Don Campaniello
Illustrator: Giovanna Pierce

Previously published as *The Path to Inner Harmony*

1 3 5 7 9 10 8 6 4 2

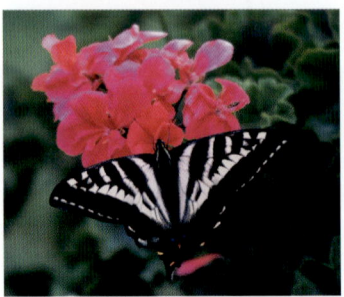

contents

introduction 6

alexander technique 12

t'ai chi 30

yoga stretches 66

meditation 82

index 94

tranquillity
gentleness balance
simplicity

introduction

There are many keys to tuning into yourself, the self that is healthy and alert, that can relax and stay calm, that sails confidently through interviews, and that knows when to step out of everyday life and enter an inner world of harmony and meditation. The secret of success starts within, knowing how to build up a strong, confident you that is in touch not just with the world out there, but your own private world of spiritual quiet. In the following pages the Alexander technique, t'ai chi, yoga, and the art of meditation all bring special ingredients to help you understand your own being, and achieve greater harmony in yourself.

inner harmony

Peace, calm and tranquillity; pressure, strife and conflict – the choice is simple. There is usually too much stress and too little peace, it is peace that we seek. From the pressurized environment of the office, or the demands of children at home, or a combination of the two, it can seem hard to find space and time for ourselves. For just a few moments of serenity, most of us would give almost anything. We would also find that our health would improve quite dramatically. Health is more than just not being ill, health is a positive, life-affirming and harmonious experience. To create this we need to balance our lives, to co-ordinate the three different aspects of our whole selves; the physical with the mental and the spiritual.

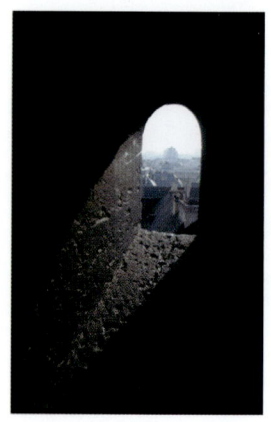

The majority of people spend much of their time in the "mental" sphere – using their intellectual capabilities to solve problems and deal with crises. Then, at the end of the day exhaustion ensues. All this can be simply remedied by balancing the different aspects of our lives. When we have balance we have harmony within. When we have inner harmony, we can hear that part of ourselves that is wise, knows what we need for health and guides us in times of difficulty. This book will help you to find ways to take time for yourself to create an oasis of calm, one in which you can relax and thrive. The ways to find this tranquillity are many; just as there are many aspects of the whole person, so there

are different approaches to achieving unity. In this book four different methods are described, ranging from those that concentrate on achieving inner harmony through almost purely physical means, to those that employ control of the mind and those that combine the physical with the mental – the Alexander technique, t'ai chi, yoga and meditation.

All these therapies and exercises are paths to inner harmony and are essentially holistic, which means that if you are not feeling well, then the whole of you is treated. You are not regarded as a production-line car that needs a quick-fix new spare part in the engine. You are seen as unique, a special integrated being in which every aspect needs to be balanced. Each part of you is considered to be equally important.

introduction

gentleness
simplicity

Together or individually, these gentle arts can quickly become a part of your daily life and aim to make you well and happy, which means that when you do suffer any kind of set-back, you are better able to cope, and should recover that bit more quickly. It is therefore important that you learn to make time to practise your favoured technique several times a day, and to adopt its principles in whatever you do. The techniques are not like special weapons that you deploy on specific occasions, but are a subtle and specific lifestyle. They do not involve any major changes at all though. People may not notice anything obviously different about you, but they will sense an air of calmness and of being in control, and of standing tall with grace and purpose (not slouching with a poor posture). It is the kind of fine tuning that can turn someone from being just noticeable to someone quite remarkable. Learning how to care and look after yourself means that you will be that much better at helping to care for others.

It is important to gain a fresh perspective on your life, demanding deadlines and schedules are not the be-all and end-all. It is important to take a little time off, otherwise you will become nervous and exhausted, a state from which it is hard to remove yourself. Remember that it is all right to make and value quiet moments, times when you can recognize and get in touch, not with the world out there, but the one inside. It will benefit not just your own well-being, but also those that are demanding work from you.

The therapies described here are excellent ways of reintroducing our modern hectic selves to the inner ones that may have been neglected. When you become a little skilled at any of them it is possible to reach simple, but wonderful inner states of calm, and you will realize exactly what you have been missing. For many, such a realization is a startling revelation that the most important thing in life is not acquiring more possessions, building extra rooms on to houses, or raising your personal profile, but just quietly "being", of reaching into yourself and finding that calming, magical privacy.

peacefulness
serenity
calmness

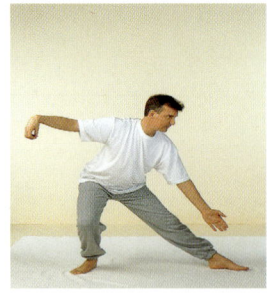

If you are particularly prone to stress and lead a demanding life, then the Alexander technique will keep you on track and help you stay focused and relaxed. This technique works in two ways – as a corrective and as a preventative measure. When we are feeling stressed, the body tenses its muscles, affecting our posture, nervous system and blood supply to important parts of our body. Overall, the mental pressures translate into physical discomforts that can quickly lead to illness – even simple poor posture can drain our energy. The Alexander technique teaches us, or reminds us of, our correct and natural poise, and this often means that you have just a little more energy which makes you better able to cope with unexpected problems, such as those at work, which may require immediate solutions. Where others may panic and suffer, you won't.

The Alexander technique is very practical and sensible. It includes advice such as how to stand properly, with every part of your body in correct alignment, or the value of lying down for 20 minutes a day to improve the head-neck-back relationship. It also teaches the use of special positions such as the "monkey" (with the legs slightly bent and hands by the knees) when doing anything strenuous, from washing the car to making a bed. The Alexander technique is easily integrated into our everyday life, helping to establish and strengthen our psycho-physical unity.

T'ai chi is a gentle, or "soft", martial art. On first glance it appears to be a purely physical pastime, but in fact it is an exceptional means of going deep inside ourselves and of gaining inner harmony. It is perfect for someone who has trouble trying to quieten their thoughts. T'ai chi emphasizes patience and relaxation and strength within softness. It improves all-round balance and posture, and imbues you with a sense of gentleness, giving you inner calm and strength, and above all balancing your Yin and Yang (the body's two complementary opposing forces).

Learning t'ai chi is a bit like learning ballet steps, except that the body does not have to make sudden leaps and twists, but learns how to flow and revolve with extraordinary grace and precision. This involves improving your ability to concentrate deeply. Initially it seems quite impossible to move through scores of set sequences inanything approaching a free-flowing style, yet after a few sessions, what seems strange and new suddenly feels totally natural. From being self-conscious and slightly awkward you will slip almost subconsciously into these wonderful trance-like movements. Watching an experienced practitioner of t'ai chi is a little like a hypnotic experience, as they withdraw deep inside themselves and yet are totally aware of that which is outside – they seem to be in some spiritual place.

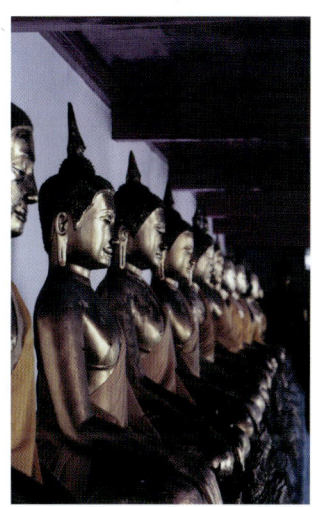

Yoga is best known as a physical exercise, though it is in fact a whole way of life covering everything from diet and spiritual matters to the well-known physical discipline. The principal effects of yoga are to stretch the body, re-aligning it and removing stressful awkward tensions, and of imparting the easy effortless qualities of a cat that combines grace with being alert. The yoga postures chosen here are essentially stretching movements which can be used at home, at work, or even on the bus. The postures sluice away stress, and leave the body and mind fresh and calm. You will often be aware of quite dramatic and uplifting effects, helping you feel well in body, mind and spirit.

The effects of meditation are very similar to yoga, except that the emphasis is on the mental: sitting and relaxing with a calm, controlled and focused mind, rather than learning certain movements and exercises. It is an exceptional way of side-stepping the rigours of daily life, and of briefly entering another world where friction and disturbance do not exist; only you, only being. Simply and quietly you will enter a state of deep relaxation, deeper than you may have experienced before.

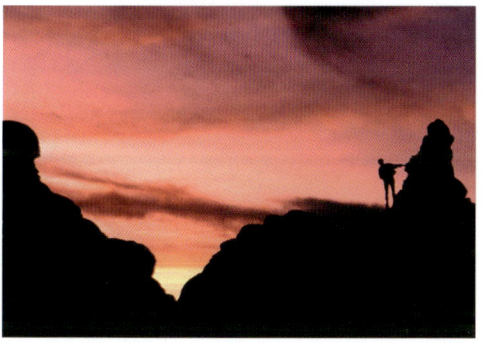

At different times you may favour one method over another, and the techniques here suit all different situations. You will find that you benefit in so many ways – you will appreciate small things more, be able to see the bigger picture, seemingly have more time, you will feel more confident and alive. You will experience peace and inner harmony, greater than you have ever known.

gentleness

alexander technique

People tend to associate the Alexander technique with relaxation, alternative medicine, body massage and with "posture". Yet it is actually much more than that.

One way towards a clearer understanding of the technique is to begin by stating what it is not. The Alexander technique does not train its teachers to make a medical diagnosis of their students, nor does it focus on any division between the mind and body. The technique believes in the indivisibility of the two and in their psycho-physical unity. Above all, the technique's main objective is to encourage people to use themselves, their bodies and minds more effectively in their day-to-day lives.

The technique's preventive role is an efficient tool which maintains tone and general well-being. It also helps to improve posture and relieve related pain. In fact it can assist people with stress-related illnesses such as respiratory and gastro-intestinal problems, as well as psychosomatic conditions. It can help those who suffer from psychological distress, such as depression, as well as facilitating recovery from accidents and injuries. The technique can even assist people with mechanical problems, such as frozen shoulder, tennis elbow and arthritis. Above all, it helps promote muscle tone and general well-being while encouraging poise and flexibility. The technique aids the well in addition to those with ailments.

the alexander technique principles

Once you start studying the technique, it quickly becomes clear that it helps you in all kinds of ways that other alternative remedies do not. That is not because it is superior, but because of its key agenda. As shown here, it helps us focus on our minds and bodies in new ways, and on aspects of our being that we might take for granted. The technique gets us back to basics.

Primary Control

"Misuse" occurs by contracting the muscles of the neck and pulling the head back and down into the shoulders. This has the twin effect of actually compressing the spine and narrowing and shortening the stature, creating tensions throughout the body. It is definitely something to be avoided.

Frederick Matthias Alexander discovered that the relationship between the head, the neck and the back, or "primary control", mechanically controlled movement and co-ordination in the whole body. To make ourselves aware of this consciously in our daily activities is the basis of good use.

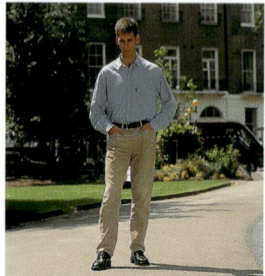

See how this model is misusing himself. He is leaning over to the right, shortening and creating an imbalance in his body.

Inhibition

In its psychological-physiological sense, inhibition means a fast-moving yet natural control of your reactions, suppressing and smothering any possible spontaneity.

However, Alexander discovered that if he managed to stop himself from behaving in his habitual way, he could choose how he wished to respond to a stimulus. If someone rings the doorbell, your immediate response may be to go straight to the door. In doing so, you will be responding habitually. If you stop yourself from responding automatically, you then choose exactly how you will approach the door with the minimum effort.

Concepts

The concept of end-gaining is extremely important in the work of Alexander technique teachers. Alexander realized that the habits he was encountering were far more deep-rooted and powerful than he had at first thought. The most serious of these was the tendency to try to react impulsively – end-gaining. End-gaining means reacting immediately and too quickly to a stimulus, without thinking. You respond by wanting something to happen, and become interested in the end result instead of being in the present. A typical example is if you are going to be late for an appointment and start to worry about the consequences. You get worked up during this process, forgetting that you might be sitting on a train, and that things are happening around you. In effect you are letting your thoughts take the situation into the future, instead of being in the "here and now", in the present.

Cutting yourself off from your environment has inevitable consequences for body positioning. It tends to lead to a pulling back of the head, a rounding of the back, a tightening of the legs and a loss of connection between the arms and the back. The gaze becomes fixed, the breath held. Essentially, the whole person is affected, both in mind and in body.

Alexander suggests you should use your "means-whereby". To put Alexander's conclusion into context, if we accept that we cannot change circumstances, we can change our approach to our bodies and allow ourselves to experience the new. It is then possible to learn to be in the moment rather than the past or the future, and to maintain a sense of inner balance and unity.

Direction

Directions are signals given by the brain to parts of the body prior to or during physical action. It is possible to alter these signals to promote a positive change. You will find that the combination of direction and inhibition enables one to transform habitual ways of moving and eliminate old patterns of misuse.

Note how this model is walking. Her head, neck and back are all correctly aligned. Her arms are free to move in a relaxed way.

Natural Poise

Nothing is more elegant and enviable than someone with perfect poise. It is something most of us have when young, but sadly it can be quickly lost to laziness and bad postural habits. In fact, it is quite easy to be totally unaware just how bad our posture is. At various times during the day it is worth freezing your movements, and taking a good look at yourself. You will be surprised at how often you fall well short of the ideal. Sitting at work is probably the one situation when your back is almost always wrongly positioned, becoming increasingly hunched, tense and stiff. Once you have ascertained exactly when and how you are going wrong, you can start putting matters right. If in any doubt, just look at young children. They instinctively know how to move gracefully and effortlessly without strain. That is something we should all try to emulate.

This child carries his toy close to his body, allowing it to lengthen and relax. This ensures good nervous energy and blood flow and allows full expansion of the lungs for breathing.

Primary Directions
- Think of freeing the neck.
- Let the head go forward and up.
- Let the back lengthen and widen.

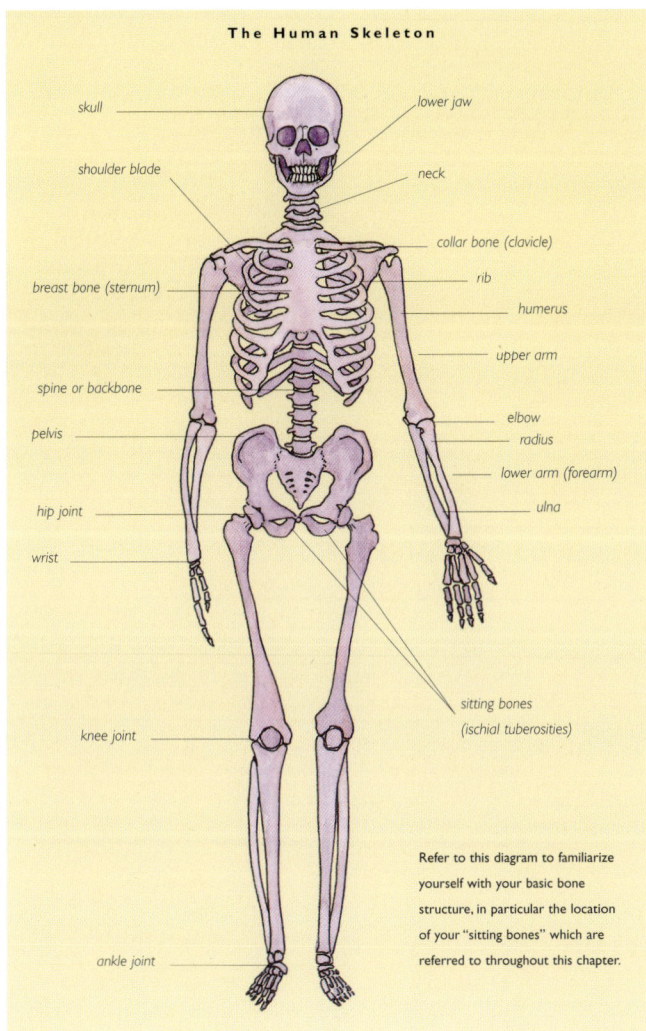

The Human Skeleton

skull — lower jaw — shoulder blade — neck — collar bone (clavicle) — rib — breast bone (sternum) — humerus — upper arm — spine or backbone — elbow — radius — pelvis — lower arm (forearm) — ulna — hip joint — wrist — sitting bones (ischial tuberosities) — knee joint — ankle joint

Refer to this diagram to familiarize yourself with your basic bone structure, in particular the location of your "sitting bones" which are referred to throughout this chapter.

Note how this child is using his joints to squat, and how he simultaneously holds the plastic bag quite effortlessly.

"Possession of property ... a means to happiness not an end."
Thomas Jefferson

putting the alexander technique into practice

A certain, rightful degree of commitment is paramount during a course of lessons because the older and more set in your ways you are, the longer it can take to change, to release unnecessary muscular tension, and to re-educate the system. Success, however, is not hard to achieve but note that it will not happen overnight, and that some slight pitfalls are always going to be inevitable, so do not be put off.

For example, you may well find yourself trying to do the directions as a routine mechanical exercise when in reality success lies in the power of the body and mind uniting as one, and in the power to think about what you are doing. Do not imagine there are any short cuts, there are not. There is also the distinct possibility that you might be tempted to give up out of sheer frustration because your time scale is too unrealistically short and limiting, and you have not allowed sufficient time for a significant, quantifiable improvement. Do not be hard on yourself, and do not imagine that you can become an expert in a ridiculously short space of time. The technique deserves more respect.

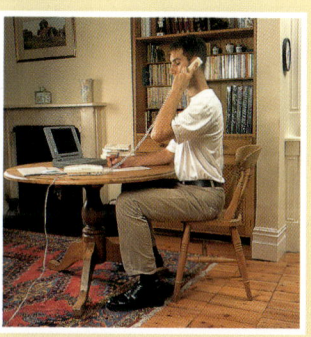

What therefore follows is the identification of the main procedures that we use most often in daily life, the areas that most concern us. In fact, the use of the word "procedure" is quite deliberate because it totally avoids the suggestion of a mind-body split and maintains a sense of psycho-physical unity. The emphasis throughout is on the means of achieving these procedures, but with the minimum of muscular tension and effort. Many students have said that a course of lessons in the technique could be compared to learning to drive or learning a new language. Dedication and determination are a sure basis for total success.

use of the eyes

If you want to know something about someone, just look straight into their eyes. They reveal an amazing amount about their current frame of mind. You can easily spot the depressed, dull and lifeless by their deadpan, almost one-dimensional eyes; the totally alert looking for a lively reply; the sad; the plaintive; the cheeky; and the happy. The technique reminds you how to stay lively and alert, and in touch with the rest of the world.

STAYING ALERT

If you observe people when they are either standing or walking, they often seem to be completely locked in a private world of their own, totally unaware of their own surroundings. They have stopped communicating with that is out there. When the gaze is fixed, the breathing also tends to suffer. It becomes rather restricted and there is less freedom in the body. The gaze should therefore be directed towards the outside world, taking in information so that you are not exclusively concentrating on what is happening within.

One of the strongest habits that a teacher perceives is the tendency of certain pupils to look down, not with their eyes, but by a general collapsing motion from the neck. This is the result of a fundamental misunderstanding of the alignment of the head, the neck and the back, and the position of the joints in the body.

Note how the models in this sequence of photographs (*below*) are using their eyes. Which do you think is the correct position? Can there be any doubt?.

"It's no good shutting your eyes if you're crossing a busy road."
F. M. Alexander

Here children are using their eyes to look at their toys. They have not disturbed the alignment between their heads, their necks and their backs, thus maintaining their good use.

In this position, the model is breaking the alignment between her head, her neck and her back as she looks down, thus using her neck inappropriately.

Note how the model is correctly aligned. She is maintaining her length and her width. Her eyes are alert and taking in her surroundings.

Here the model is breaking at the neckline and pulling her head back to look up, disturbing the alignment between her head, neck and back.

the semi-supine position

Standing for long periods easily compresses the spine. Lying down in a semi-supine position is a way of alleviating unnecessary tensions in the muscles and joints, and should be practised every day for at least 20 minutes. It encourages a better awareness of the head-neck-back relationship. This position does not necessarily need monitoring by a teacher, and it also gives you much needed time for yourself.

THE POSITION

Try to keep your eyes alert and open. It is preferable to avoid closing them because you will probably find it quite difficult not to fall asleep, which is definitely not the point of the exercise!

During your daily 20-minute session try and give yourself the time to practise some sharp, well directed thoughts to avoid your mind from wandering and spreading out, covering other possible important issues. This session can also encourage you to put into practice your excellent skills of observation. A good practice is to go over the primary directions, and to notice if you are aware of any tension in your body and to address it without trying to correct it. That is the secret of success.

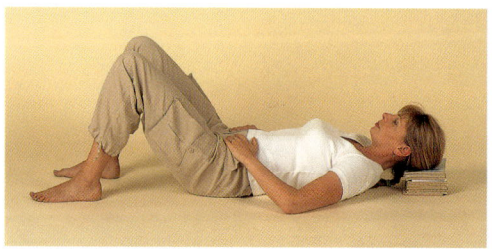

Books are used to support the head. If you have too many, however, your chin will drop and you will feel pressure on your throat.

Correspondingly, if you do not have enough books your head will tilt back and will not be properly supported.

MOVING INTO THE SEMI-SUPINE

It is preferable to lie down on a hard, carpeted surface or alternatively on a rug on the floor. Avoid beds as they will not offer you adequate support. The number of books you need will depend on their thickness, and will also vary from person to person.

To lie down on the floor, place the books far enough behind you to give enough space for the whole of your torso and your bottom. When sitting, you can place your hands palms down on the floor behind you to help you lower your back. Take care not to stiffen the arms or to hold your breath in the process. To get up, it is preferable to roll over to one side, leading with your eyes rather than your head, and following with your torso and legs. Then place the free hand flat on the floor and go on to all fours. Be careful to maintain the alignment between your head, your neck and your back and not to hold your breath. Walk your hands back so that you move your bottom back towards your heels.

Make sure that your legs are about hip-width apart and that your knees are directed towards the ceiling.

If your knees are falling out, you will probably lose the contact between the inner side of your foot and the floor.

sitting and standing

Correct posture is as much about what is right as what is wrong. It is vital that you know what to do, and what not to do. It is easy to start out with correct posture, but fall into bad habits. You must know when to correct yourself. Remember to keep a straight alignment between head, neck and back, and to keep your legs hip-width apart with knees pointing forward, in the same direction as your feet.

SITTING

Correct: think of the shoulders going away from each other.

Incorrect: rounded shoulders and feet wrapped around chair legs.

Incorrect: arching the back, folding legs and leaning to one side.

FROM SITTING TO STANDING

It is well worth practising this basic technique several times to perfect it. You will be surprised how ingrained bad habits are. Start by placing your legs about hip-width apart. Avoid pushing firmly up with them; that is not the object. Also, make sure that your feet are flat and are not placed so far forwards that coming up to stand is in any way difficult. Finally, remember to lead with the head; that is the key to getting this technique right.

1 Here the model is relaxed, feet apart, hands resting comfortably, ready to go into the standing position.

2 As she stands she has managed to keep the correct alignment between her head, neck and back.

3 Having hinged from the hip, sending her knees forwards and away over her feet, she is now properly upright.

alexander technique 21

reaching and handling

It is impossible to avoid two basic movements, reaching and handling. Yet how many of us know how to do them properly, according to the Alexander technique? Reaching means keeping the alignment between the head, neck and back, whether you are low down or standing up. If you are indeed squatting, it is important that you allow your hand to lead your movement. Let everything else follow behind.

HANDLING

See how the model's weight is balanced over the feet, and how she is allowing her hand to lead her wrist and arm.

Here, the legs are straight and the head is pulled back, causing a lot of strain on the neck, and the shoulders are tense.

See how the arms remain well connected to the shoulder blades and back. Also, there is no tension in the arms and wrists.

GOING UP ON TIPTOES

When going on tiptoes correctly, the weight that is placed on the middle of the feet when standing is placed on the balls of the feet, as the head leads the body forwards and upwards. It is important to maintain the alignment between the head, the neck and the back. The breath is not held, and the eyes are alert.

Look at how this model is going on tiptoes to enable her hand to lead her arm to close the window.

Note how the model is well poised and correctly aligned. There is no undue stress on the body.

Here the head contraction is severe. The model is holding his breath, causing unnecessary tension in the body.

"monkey" or bending

The position known as the "monkey" enables us to move with more flexibility in our daily activities. It is a useful means of moving from standing to sitting or squatting, as well as helping with lifting, picking things up, working at a desk, washing, ironing, and participating in sports such as skiing and golf. The "monkey" respects the relationship between the head, neck and back.

THE POSITION

The "monkey" position might sound tricky, but it really is not. Try it slowly, see how it works, then try it again at a more natural speed. It basically involves the head moving forwards and up, and then the knees moving forwards and away over the feet to counterbalance the bottom going back over the heels, enabling the arms to move freely. It is also important to remember that when you go into "monkey" you must review your primary directions. What is more, stay alert at all times, and avoid fixing your gaze or holding your breath. Such moves will quickly undermine the marvellous effects of the "monkey".

To be more precise then, stand with your legs hip-width apart, with the feet slightly turned outwards. Your weight should be evenly distributed, neither too far forwards nor too far back on your feet. To start going into the "monkey", allow the knees to bend slightly over your feet as you tilt forwards from your hip joints, making sure your head, your neck and your back are aligned. Avoid collapsing over yourself!

One final point is to make sure you think of widening and lengthening your back as you widen across the shoulder girdle, to allow free movement and your arms to hang freely. This extra tip will ensure you enjoy the full effect of "the monkey".

This model is in the correct "monkey" position. Her head, her neck and her back are aligned. Her knees are bent forward and away from her hips.

When going into the "monkey" avoid retracting the head back and down into the spine. Note how the model has rounded her shoulders and pulled in her knees.

Here the model is not bending her knees as she bends forwards. Her back is collapsed over her body, and her legs are straight and braced.

everyday situations

In everyday situations it is important to pause before reacting, to make sure you are so positioned that you do not misuse yourself. The more aware you are, the more likely you will encourage muscular release through your whole system. Equally, the more at peace you are, the easier it is to apply the principles of the Alexander technique. The following excellent examples show how the "monkey" can keep you healthy.

Note how the model's back is correctly aligned, keeping to the head-neck-back principle. See how she is using her joints and allowing her widening arms to handle the dish.

How things can go wrong. Here the model has started pulling her head back. Also, her back is rounded, her legs are braced and her arms have become much too tense.

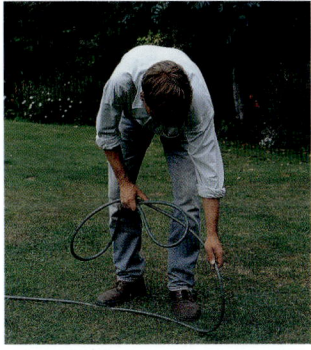

In this highly incorrect stance, the man is collapsing from his waist down as he begins works in the garden. His shoulders are far too rounded, and his head is being pulled back.

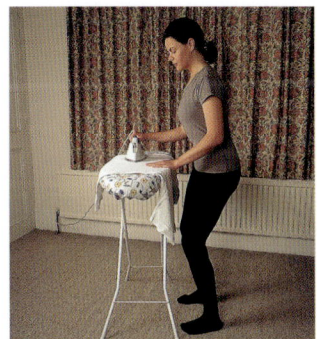

In this correct procedure, the model is neatly poised and balanced, and she is well aligned to begin her ironing. Her hand, wrist and arm are also free as she holds the iron. The other crucial point to note is how she is widening across her upper arms. It is clear that she looks balanced and feels alert.

See how the model is using the whole of his back quite correctly. He is sensibly allowing his weight to come back on to his heels, and his knees go forwards and away over his feet.

An example of how not to do it. Here he is completely out of alignment. You can sense it is not right, but why? He is actually pulling his head back, rounding the back, and holding in the arms. This position is entirely the result of bad habits. Without the Alexander technique, he would never know how to right this.

"lunge monkey"

The "lunge monkey" is similar to the "monkey" because the knees go forwards and away, and the torso tilts slightly forwards from the hip joints. Also, one foot is placed behind the other, and the legs are placed hip-width apart, enabling you to balance the upper part of your body on to the forward or the back leg whenever the need arises. In this way, your weight is placed forwards or backwards according to your activity.

BENDING

The "lunge monkey" is extremely useful when you need to lift something heavy from the floor; when you need to move an object from one side of a surface to another, for example during cooking; or when you need to push or pull something rather heavy into place.

When you adapt the "lunge monkey" it is important to remember to keep your head, your neck and your back correctly aligned. The legs must be hip-width apart, with the arms hanging freely on either side of your torso.

Also, allow your weight to move to the right on to the right foot (or to the left, as the situation demands). If moving to the left, reverse the instructions.

See how the model has collapsed badly from the waist down. Her shoulders are rounded, the legs are straight and the knees are braced, causing tension.

Observe how the model has gone into the "lunge monkey". Her head, neck and back are neatly aligned, and her knees are going forward away from her hips.

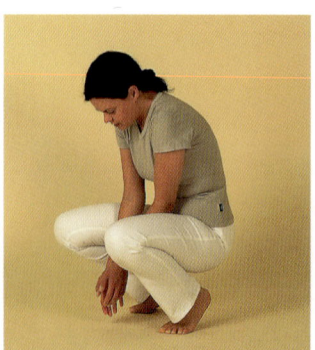

Note how the model has completely lost the correct alignment with her back as she squats. Her head has dropped, and her shoulders are hunched and rounded. Furthermore, she looks ill at ease and uncomfortable. There is no poise or grace. This position is definitely one to avoid.

In this correct procedure, observe how the model's head, neck and back are correctly aligned. Her shoulders are widening across her upper arms. She looks well balanced, and fully in control of her movements. Also note how her heels are tucked in under the bottom. The position is also easy to get into.

SQUATTING

In Western societies most people find it difficult to squat in their everyday lives. Young children have very little difficulty in doing so, but as we grow older we lose the necessary flexibility to squat as our joints become less mobile.

A low "monkey" or semi-squat is the best way that an Alexander teacher can re-introduce a student to squatting over a series of lessons. To squat, follow the same guidelines as for the "monkey", but with a wider stance. Remember to maintain the alignment between the head, the neck and the back, and to allow the joints in the hips, the knees and the ankles to be free. As you go into a deeper squat you might find that your heels come off the ground. This does not present a problem as far as the technique is concerned, so long as you keep your balance. As a general rule, go only as far as you feel comfortable.

alexander technique

the technique in the home

The key point to note about the Alexander technique is that it is not an abstract theory that you can apply when the mood takes you. It is a specific, practical everyday guide that will help you enormously whether you are bending, squatting, lifting or carrying. It gives you terrific control whatever you are doing, injecting extra confidence that will keep you alert and relaxed.

BENDING

Note how the model is tilted forwards to get a greater range of movement. His arms are free, supported by his back.

Now he is incorrectly bending forwards from the waist. His legs are braced, and his head is pulled back.

Here the model has aligned herself nicely to make the bed. Her legs are bent, creating a greater range of movement.

SQUATTING

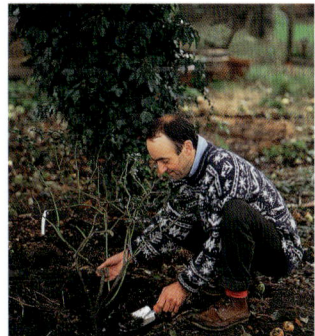

This model is lunge squatting to brush up dirt from the floor. She has maintained her good use, giving herself a maximum range of movement. She looks good and feels good.

Here, in an incorrect example of how you should sweep the floor, the model is badly restricting his range of movement. He is quite clearly unbalanced, and feels totally uncomfortable.

Note how this man is squatting sensibly to plant a rose bush in his garden. By placing himself at the same level as the rose, he is allowing himself a greater range of movement.

lifting and carrying

A lot of back pain is the result of lifting heavy weights. To avoid back strain, stand near to the load by placing your feet either side of it, and maintain the alignment between head, neck and back. Go into the "monkey" or "lunge monkey" and squat. Then bend your arms so that your elbows are close to your body. Make sure that you widen out across the upper arms, and avoid tension in the arms and wrists.

LIFTING

1 Once you are holding the load as closely to your body as you can, come out of a squat or lunge squat into a "monkey" before standing.

2 Lift the weight in a flowing action, that does not jar or suddenly pull against the back. If the weight proves too heavy, it is easy to bend and put it down.

3 To place the load back on the ground, reverse the process and apply the same principles, making sure that your head, neck and back are aligned.

CARRYING

Here the model is carrying all her shopping bags in one hand, creating an imbalance as she is pulled down to the left. She is raising her right shoulder in an attempt to support her handbag.

This model is carrying her shopping bags sensibly and correctly so that they are evenly distributed on both sides. She is well balanced and able to walk freely. She looks content.

Look at the excellent way this mother is carrying her child. Her weight is evenly distributed and she is holding the child close to her body, firmly supporting his upper and lower body.

daily routines

The most surprising point about the Alexander technique is that it is not just for big, set piece movements such as lifting heavy weights, when doing it incorrectly can obviously lead to back problems. The technique even extends to the minutiae of life, routines that we completely take for granted, such as eating, drinking, and driving. If you had always wondered how they should be done, read on. These tips will make all the difference.

EATING AND DRINKING

If you are standing upright while you are drinking remember that you still need to be fully alert at all times. Therefore, make sure that you do not fix your gaze rigidly and thereby lose all communication and contact with the outside world. You also need to ensure that your head leads you away from your heels (see the section on Standing for further guidance). You will find that your shoulder girdle brings mobility to your arms, and that the pelvis provides stability which simultaneously facilitates mobility in your legs.

The very same principles also apply to eating. Whether you are going to eat something from your hand or use a fork, it is all too easy to forget your posture completely. Remember that you should not totally focus on the matter in hand, but that you must also consider your stance, alertness and poise.

Avoid gripping or clutching your glass. Be aware of the connection with your arm, which links to your back and then into your heels. As you raise the cup to your lips, bring your weight back on to the heels, so as not to pull in your lower back. Also, bring the glass to the lips, rather than leaning down into it.

Take some time to consider how you are seated at the table and then bring the food up to your mouth, rather than the reverse. Your feet should be correctly positioned on the floor. You should also be aware of both your sitting bones, and how your back should be lengthening and widening. This position also aids digestion.

DRIVING

Most of the problems experienced by drivers are due to fixed postures, long journeys and poor seating support.

Too many people who spend huge amounts of time driving find themselves constricted by the position of the steering wheel and the pedals. Such a cramped environment is bound to lead to stress and strain on the back, and equally on the arms and legs.

When choosing a car take time to see whether the seat is firm and supportive. If you already own a car and it does not have a lumbar support adjustment, you can use a wedge-shaped cushion to give you adequate support in the lumbar area and the pelvis. It makes a vital difference.

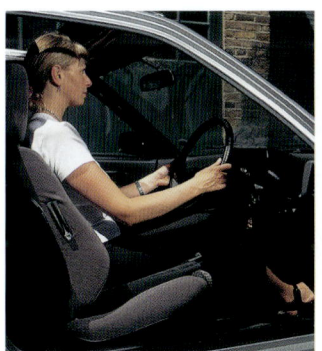

You should be able to reach the pedals quite easily. A wedge-shaped cushion is extremely useful to avoid a poor, slumping position.

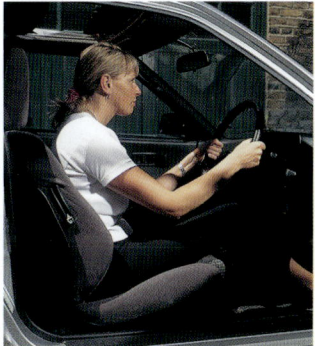

See how the model is badly collapsing forward, how the neck is being strained and the arms are rigidly tense. Such a position will cause lots of discomfort.

office work

Before reading it is important to spend some time considering exactly how you are going to sit in order to avoid badly slumping, which is very easy to do, especially in a big old comfortable armchair. Once you get drawn into what you are reading it is virtually certain that you will completely forget about your posture. It is vitally important that you do not end up creating all kinds of stresses and strains in your body.

READING AND WRITING

When you are sitting at your desk or at a table, it is important that you adjust your chair in such a way that your lower arms and hands can be placed on the surface of your table or desk at a right angle. If your chair is too close you are likely to end up lifting your shoulders to adjust your arms. If your chair is too high, you will probably find that you start slumping. You must also avoid crossing your legs, and do make sure that your feet remain comfortably flat on the floor.

A useful trick when reading is to use a sloping board to avoid slumping over your desk or table.

Note how the model is holding her body badly with her arm, and how her legs are folded, offering no support.

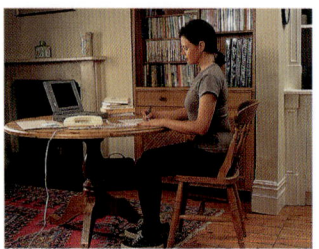

Keep the alignment between your head, your neck and your back.

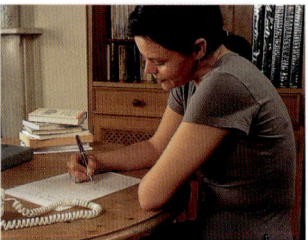

This model is firmly gripping the pen, causing tension in her wrist and hand.

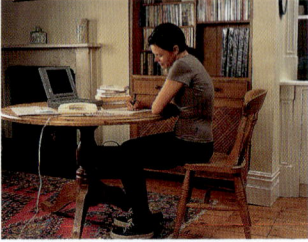

Here the model is tensing her wrist, hand and arm, restricting her movement.

DESKWORK

An increasing number of people are complaining of neck and shoulder tension, wrist problems and back pain resulting from their working environment. Some cases are directly linked to badly designed furniture, awkward or unfavourable sitting positions and immobility. In other instances, although chairs and work surfaces are good, the posture is poor. You must therefore remember your primary directions: the head, neck and back should be aligned, and the head should be lengthening away from the sitting bones.

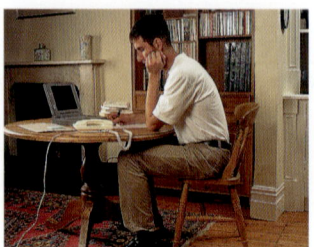

How not to do it. See how the model is slumping badly, causing unnecessary tension in the spine, so weakening the muscles surrounding the torso.

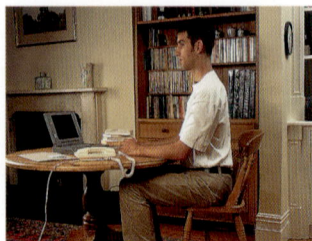

Here the spine is correctly aligned, and the head is poised gracefully above the neck. The feet are well placed on the floor, nicely apart.

office equipment

The office is not what it used to be. It now offers amazing improvements in high-tech equipment, but also plenty of opportunities for repetitive strain injury, aching backs and tense necks. The temptation is to spend far too long in one awkward position. So always be aware of what you are doing, how long it will take, and the best position you need to adopt. Such awareness makes all the difference between a good and bad day.

MOBILE PHONE USE

Observe Yourself When the Telephone Rings

Do you snatch and grab it? Or do you try to give yourself some time before you pick up the receiver? Next time the telephone rings, stop and go over your primary directions. Make sure that you bring the receiver up to your ear rather than suddenly leaning down towards it, thus compromising your position.

Here the model is pulling her head down wrongly towards her mobile phone to talk, and slouching.

In this example the model has maintained her balance throughout her body. She looks poised and relaxed.

WORKING AT A COMPUTER

If you are working at a computer or portable computer, use your eyes to look down towards it. Avoid lurching at the neck as you will lose the correct alignment with your back.

Here the model badly collapses over her computer. She has lost the correct alignment between her hands, her wrists and her lower arms. Her shoulders are far too hunched.

Here the model is incorrectly holding in her wrist, arms and shoulders, causing unnecessary strain and discomfort. She will soon feel very uncomfortable, and have to adopt a new position.

t'ai chi

T'ai chi ch'uan is an ancient form of slow, graceful and rhythmic exercise which originated in China, where it is still extremely popular, often being performed in public parks in the fresh morning air. It has its roots in Taoist philosophy. The movements of the t'ai chi form gently tone and strengthen the organs and muscles, improve circulation and posture, and relax both mind and body. Its name translates as "supreme ultimate fist", but this is not its true meaning. "Strength within softness", "poetry in motion" and "moving harmony" all come closer to expressing the spirit of t'ai chi.

T'ai chi has been variously described as a system of health, medicine, physical co-ordination, relaxation, self-defence and consciousness raising, as well as a means of exercise and self-development. It is all these things. The style shown here is the Yang-style short form, as developed by Professor Cheng Man-Ch'ing, which is the one most practised in the West.

Unlike the "hard" martial arts which rely on force and speed, t'ai chi is "soft" or "internal". Its emphasis lies in the yielding aspect of nature when overcoming the hard – like the waterfall which eventually wears away the rock beneath. It teaches patience and relaxation, and fosters an understanding of the co-ordination of mind, body and spirit. It is the perfect antidote to the stresses and strains of today's modern lifestyles.

t'ai chi for health or self defence

If you simply want to go out and strike a pose, jumping about like Bruce Lee, t'ai chi is not for you. It is a very serious, highly regarded ancient technique that has two major qualities. It improves your health, and teaches you how to overcome stronger hostile forces when you are under attack. The most amazing part of t'ai chi is the way its movements are almost balletic.

The Benefits of T'ai Chi

Although t'ai chi can eventually be used in self-defence, and most classes do incorporate some of its practical applications, it is initially practised mainly for its health-giving benefits. It is particularly useful for increasing alertness and body awareness, and for developing concentration and sensitivity. It helps with balance and posture, and enhances a sense of "groundedness". However, all the postures can also be used when defending yourself against an attack by an opponent. Its gentleness and subtlety do not preclude its use as a very effective form of self-defence.

It is not easy to separate the physical and mental aspects of t'ai chi, as they are closely interrelated. In Chinese medicine, the interdependence of mind, body and spirit is seen as integral to well-being.

The ancient art of t'ai chi instills enormous grace and confidence.

The Theory of T'ai Chi

Like music, t'ai chi cannot be appreciated purely on an intellectual level. It also has an enormous spiritual side, and when you watch any highly experienced t'ai chi practitioners you will see how they are almost in a kind of trance, in a separate world where they cannot be touched. Correctly done, it is quite hypnotic.

For now, we must look at some of the concepts that are fundamental to the martial arts, as well as to medicine and philosophy. Although these disciplines are all treated quite separately by those in the West, they are all inseparable in the Eastern view. From thousands of years of close observation of patterns of energy, the Chinese successfully evolved a way of life that actually ropes all three ingredients together.

Chi

Chi is the prime driving force of human life, the spark behind thought, creativity and growth which maintains and nurtures us. It can be felt as movement of energy in the body, like the ceaseless flow of an electrical current. Chi flows through the body along channels called meridians.

The Tan Tien

The Chi is stored in the Tan Tien. This is an area about the size of a golf ball, located four finger-widths below the navel, and about one-third of the way from the front to the back of the body. It is the centre of gravity of the body, and in t'ai chi all movement emanates from it. Try to let the breath and the mind sink to the Tan Tien.

Yin and Yang

Yin and Yang describe the complementary yet opposing forces of nature. Their relationship has a harmony and balance: both Yin and Yang are necessary, are constantly moving and balancing each other, and this interaction creates Chi. The Chinese observed that when the balance of Yin and Yang is disrupted so too will be the body's Chi, leading to ill health.

One of the key requirements for t'ai chi is excellent balance.

warm-up exercises

Perform these exercises slowly and gently, with the mind and the breath focused in the Tan Tien. Notice any differences between the right and left sides of your body, and between the upper and lower parts. The object is gradually to enter the world of t'ai chi, and to warm up all your muscles so that you do not get any strains. The more you warm up, the better your technique will be. The movements will flow like a stream.

CIRCLING HANDS

1 Inhale and allow both hands to float upwards a comfortable distance in front of your body, palms facing downwards.

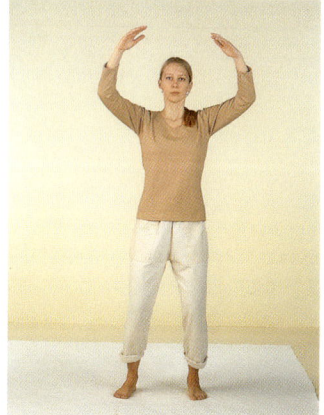

2 As your hands rise above your head, relax the wrists and begin to open the palms outwards. Begin to exhale.

3 Open out your arms to your sides. Draw your hands inwards at the bottom of the circle and smoothly begin again.

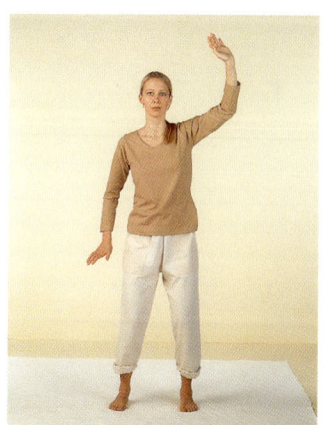

4 Inhale as your palms, facing upwards, float in front of your body. Exhale and push your right hand down by your hip and your left hand up by your temple.

5 Breathe in again, relax your palms which now turn to face each other and begin moving them towards each other in front of your body.

6 Repeat step 4 in reverse as you exhale. Breathe in again and bring your hands in front of your body in a mirror image of Step 5.

SHAKING OUT SHOULDERS, ARMS AND HANDS

1 Gently shake out any tension in your wrists and hands. Gradually work up to include your shoulders. This exercise is especially useful before, during and after long periods at a keyboard, or repetitive work with the hands.

LOOSENING SHOULDERS

1 Make increasing circles with one shoulder. Change direction and decrease the size of the circles. Repeat for the other shoulder. Rotate your shoulders alternately.

ROTATING WAIST

1 Place both hands lightly on your hips. Keeping your head up, begin by spiralling your hips slowly outwards, feeling for any restriction, tightness or lack of ease. Change direction and spiral back in slowly.

KNEE ROTATIONS

1 Bring your feet together and place your palms lightly on your upper kneecaps. Feel the Chi from your palms radiating deep into your knee joints. Circle your knees clockwise several times, then change direction.

2 Keep your legs and hands in the same position. Rotate your knees in opposite directions – one circles clockwise while the other circles anti-clockwise (counter-clockwise). Change the direction of each knee and repeat the rotations.

CALF STRETCH

1 Step forward with your right foot. Keeping the heel on the floor, pull up your toes towards the knee. Drop your body forward, keeping your right leg straight. Hold for a few breaths and release. Repeat for the other leg.

FOUR-DIRECTIONAL BREATHING

1 As you inhale, bring your hands up to chest height, palms facing upwards.

2 As you exhale, turn the palms to face away and extend your arms as if pushing something away. On the next inhalation, turn your palms back to face your body, softening your arms and drawing them back in towards your chest.

3 Exhale again, turn the palms out and extend your arms out to your sides.

4 Relax and bring your arms in towards your chest as you inhale.

5 On the next exhalation turn your palms upwards and extend your arms towards the sky.

6 Inhale and let your arms descend, palms facing downwards. As your arms pass the solar plexus, exhale and push down towards the earth. Repeat this sequence several times.

ROTATING FROM THE WAIST WITH FEET FORWARD

1 Imagine a central axis from the crown of your head, dropping down through your body to a point between your feet. Rotate your body around this axis, keeping your arms relaxed.

2 As your waist turns to the left, your weight shifts on to your left leg. As it turns right, move your weight across on to your right leg. Let your arms swing naturally.

3 Repeat the sequence for about 1 minute. As you do it, try to keep each knee over its respective big toe to avoid any strain on the muscles and ligaments.

ROTATING FROM THE WAIST TURNING ON THE BALL OF THE FOOT

1 The arms follow the same movement as above, but each foot pivots in turn on the ball. Keeping your weight in your left leg, turn your waist to the right. Lift your right heel and swivel the right foot 90°.

2 As your waist returns to the centre, straighten your right foot until your feet are parallel and shoulder-width apart. Transfer your weight on to your right foot.

3 Turn your waist to the left, lift your left heel and pivot on the ball of your left foot. Repeat the sequence for about 1 minute, keeping your head up, back straight and arms and shoulders relaxed.

OPENING AND CLOSING THE CIRCLE

1 Place your hands in front of your face, palms facing away. Turn your waist slowly to the right.

2 Drop almost all your weight into your right leg and continue turning your waist, bending forwards which in turn brings your hands around in a large circular movement.

3 As your hands cross the bottom of the circle, shift your weight into your left leg. Continue to turn your waist slowly, bringing your hands up to complete the circle.

4 When your hands reach their starting-point in front of your face, repeat the sequence and continue for several more rotations.

5 Change direction gently at the bottom of the circle to repeat the sequence. This time, join your palms together lightly at the top of each circle.

6 Keep the palms together as you turn, allowing your hands to separate at the bottom. Finish the exercise by keeping your palms connected and spiralling your hands to end in front of your chest.

SHIFTING WEIGHT

ROTATING WHOLE BODY

1 Place your left foot at 45° and your right foot forward, heels shoulder-width apart. Shift your weight from one leg to the other – do not tip your pelvis forwards or backwards.

2 Let your arms swing naturally. Continue for about 1 minute, then change legs and repeat the sequence again. Feel a strong root developing through your feet into the centre of the earth.

1 Hold both arms in front of the chest, palms facing inwards, fingertips almost touching. Turn your waist and arms and shift your weight to the right. Repeat to the left.

WAVING HANDS IN CLOUDS

1 Begin with your right hand facing the Tan Tien, your left hand directly above it, facing your chest. Turn your waist to the left, shifting your weight into your left leg. Turn your palms towards each other.

2 Bring your waist back to the front. As you do so, lower your left hand until it is opposite the Tan Tien and raise your right hand to the level of your chest, with your palms facing your body.

3 Now turn your waist to the right, shift the weight across to your right leg, and turn your palms towards each other in a mirror image of Step 1. Repeat the entire sequence several times.

PUSH TO CENTRE, PUSH TO CORNER

1 Place your right foot at 45° and step forward with your left foot. Begin with all your weight on your right leg, right hand resting palm upwards on your right hip, left fingertips in line with your mouth, palm facing diagonally forwards and to the centre.

2 Bring your weight forward on to your left leg. Your right hand turns diagonally forwards as it comes to push towards the centre of your body; your left hand turns palm upwards as it draws back to rest on your left hip.

3 Shift your weight back on to your right foot, turning your waist 45° to the right. At the same time draw your right hand back to your right hip and push your left hand towards the corner until it is in line with the centre of your body, fingertips opposite your mouth. Repeat steps 1, 2 and 3 for about 1 minute.

4 Repeat the sequence in mirror image as it is shown above. Make sure that all your movements are smooth and flowing and that the weight is gently shifted between your feet.

5 Bring your weight on to your right leg. Your left hand turns diagonally forwards as it comes towards the centre of the body, your right palm turns upwards as it draws back to rest on the right hip.

6 Shift your weight to your left foot, turning your waist 45° to the left. At the same time, draw your left hand to your left hip and push your right hand to the corner. Repeat the cycle in Steps 5 and 6.

NECK ROTATIONS

1 Keep the palms of your hands in front of your chest, fingertips almost touching. Relax your shoulders and elbows. Turn your head to look over one shoulder, then the other. Repeat several times, keeping the neck movements fluid.

HIP ROTATIONS

1 Turn out your left foot and sink all your weight on to it. Draw a smooth circle with your right knee, keeping the hip movement as fluid as possible. Repeat the same rotation on the other hip.

ANKLE ROTATIONS

1 Place your left foot at 45°, bend your left knee and sink all your weight into your left leg. Lift your right foot and slowly rotate the ankle, describing a circle with your big toe. Repeat the exercise for the left ankle.

RETURN TO CENTRE

1 As you breathe in, take your hands out to the sides in front of your body, and raise them slowly in a large circle, palms facing upwards.

2 As you exhale, lower your hands in front of the centre of your body, palms facing downwards.

3 At the bottom of the circle, turn your hands outwards again to begin a new circle with the new breath.

KIDNEY MASSAGE

1 The kidneys are the most important organs, according to Chinese medicine, as they store the Chi. This massage provides gentle stimulation and helps to break down crystals of uric acid found in kidney stones. Bring your heels together at right angles, and massage around your kidneys with loose fists.

ABDOMINAL MASSAGE

1 With your heels together, massage your abdomen in a circular motion with the palms of your hands to assist and bring blood to the digestive area.

STIMULATING THE BACK OF THE NECK

1 Lift your hands to the back of your head. Flick your index and middle fingers over each other to tap the base of the occipital ridge at the back of the skull, releasing Chi up to the top of your head. Flick the back of your head about 20 times.

FEELING THE AIR

1 With your heels together and feet at right angles, inhale and let both hands float up towards your shoulders, palms facing upwards. Feel the resistance of the air on your palms.

2 As you exhale, let both hands float back down. Try to feel resistance on the backs of your hands, and the air rushing softly between your fingers.

STILLNESS WITHIN MOVEMENT

1 Bring your heels together at right angles to each other. Try to feel where your body weight naturally lies. After a few quiet moments of standing still, you can begin some t'ai chi walking, or start the form. Notice the feelings you have, especially in the Tan Tien, and carry these feelings with you into the form.

yang-style short form

After completing all the warm-up exercises, and having a moment or so quietly standing to see if you can find a point of equilibrium, a few minutes of t'ai chi walking may now follow. This is known as walking with an "empty step", rather in the manner of a cat tentatively putting out its paw before committing its full weight on to the front leg.

In fact, it is well worth studying an adult cat that is gracefully walking, or gliding forwards when it has spotted its prey. Its whole movement is one of ceaseless flow, of elegant, unforced movement when every part of its body seems to be an extension of another part, and nothing is hurried or rushed.

As you progress through the form, use the following pages as an aide-mémoire for your practice, especially for the transitions from one posture to the next. Remember to keep your movements slow and smooth, like clouds drifting gently by on a summer's day, and relax. If you worry about this new exercise, you will not succeed.

In many ways that is the key problem for the new Western practitioner. Doing these exercises initially means that you will be highly self-conscious because there is nothing like it in our culture. Yet gradually, after a few lessons, and above all after watching expert t'ai chi practitioners, it becomes clear that this is something which you can do successfully, and without having to worry about what you look like.

Once you launch into the first few movements, the rest follow, and you find that an awkward state of self-consciousness is quickly replaced by an inner calm as you become less aware of the outside world, and more aware of inner ones. The key to t'ai chi is being able to make seamless flowing moves, with the emphasis not so much on specific poses as on the linking means of getting there. Ultimately, you too may be able to go into a park in the early morning, as they do in the East, and carry out t'ai chi utterly unself-consciously, gaining spiritual refreshment.

ATTENTION, PREPARATION AND BEGINNING

1 Stand in a relaxed and upright posture, feet pointing diagonally outwards, making a right angle. Distribute your weight evenly through your body.

2 Bend your right knee and sink all your weight down through your right leg into the foot, without leaning across. Then move the "empty" left leg a shoulder-width away, with the toes pointing straight ahead.

3 Transfer 70% of your weight to your left leg, simultaneously turning your waist and therefore your whole body diagonally to the right.

4 Keeping 70% of your weight in your left leg, turn your whole body back to face the front. Bring your right foot around to the front as your waist moves. Your feet should be shoulder-width apart and parallel. Your hands also move with your body, the palms facing the ground as if resting on a cushion of air.

5 Relax your wrists and let your arms float up and away from your body. When your hands reach shoulder height, gently extend the fingertips.

6 Draw your hands back in towards your body by dropping the elbows. This penultimate posture is one of relaxed, graceful ease.

WARD OFF LEFT

7 In the final position, relax your wrists and let your hands float down the front of your body, just in front of and below the waist. The bulk of your weight is in your left leg.

1 Sink all your weight on to your left leg, and turn your body to the right, pivoting on your right heel. Imagine you are holding a large ball, with the right hand in front of the chest.

2 Sink all your weight on to your right leg, as if carrying the ball forward. Pick up your "empty" (weightless) left leg and step forwards, toes pointing to the front.

WARD OFF RIGHT

3 Turn the waist to the left, facing the front. Your left hand comes up, palm facing the chest, and the right floats down with 70% of your weight now on your left leg, as your right moves around.

1 Sink all your weight into your left leg. Turn to the right: the left palm turns face down, the right palm turns up as if both hands are again holding the large ball. The heels should be slightly apart.

2 Turn your waist to face the right-hand side and shift 70% of your weight on to your right foot, and turn your left foot to 45°. Raise your right arm so that the palm faces your chest.

ROLL BACK, PRESS AND PUSH

This posture, together with the one that follows it, "Single Whip", is also known as "Grasping the Sparrow's Tail".

1 Turn your body to the right. Point the fingertips of your right hand to the sky in a relaxed way. Your left arm moves horizontally with the fingertips almost touching the right elbow, palm facing the body. Your weight remains 70% on the right leg, 30% on the left.

2 As you turn your waist to the left, begin to shift weight to your left leg. Follow the movement of the body with your arms until your right hand is horizontal. Your left hand begins to flow down with the movement of your waist. Your weight settles on your left leg.

3 Turn your waist back to the right and let your left arm follow this movement. All your weight remains in the left leg. Bring your palm gradually across to rest against your right wrist, opposite the centre of your chest.

4 Press forward, keeping the hands in full contact. Shift 70% of your weight into your front (right) leg. Ensure that your heels are still shoulder-width apart, and that the right foot is pointing forward, and the left foot at 45°.

5 Separate your hands and sink all your weight back into your left foot. Your fingertips are now shoulder-width apart at shoulder height.

6 Move your weight forward 70% into your right leg. Your arms and hands keep the same position.

SINGLE WHIP

1 As your weight shifts back into the left leg, leave your fingers where they are in space, effectively straightening – but not locking – your arms. The palms now face down towards the ground.

2 Turn your whole body to the left and shift all your weight into your left leg. Your right heel remains on the ground while your toes turn through 120°, following the body round.

3 Sink your weight back into your right leg. Bring your left hand under the right to hold the imaginary ball in front of your body. Then form a "hook" with the fingers and thumb of your right hand.

4 Ensure all your weight is in your right leg. Bend the right knee and turn your body to the left, sending out the hook in line with, and at the same height as, your shoulder. Take an "empty" (weightless) shoulder-width step with your left foot.

5 Shift 70% of your weight on to your left leg, adjusting your right foot to 45°. Ensure that your heels are shoulder-width apart, your left hand in line with your left shoulder and your right hand hook at 90° to the rest of your body.

LIFTING HANDS

1 Place your weight on the left leg, open your hands and palms inwards, the left palm facing the right elbow. Pick up your empty right foot and place down the heel without weight, directly in front of the left heel.

WHITE CRANE SPREADS WINGS AND PUSH

2 Turn your waist to the left, your hands following the movement of your waist. Bring your right toe by your left heel, touching the ground but weightless.

3 Take an "empty" step to the right, and transfer 70% of the weight to the right foot. The left palm ends up opposite your inner right elbow. Your right arm is curved, guarding the groin, and your feet are at right angles to each other.

1 Drop all your weight into your right leg. Turn your waist to the left. As your right hand begins to rise, your left hand sweeps down in front of your left thigh.

2 Pick up your "empty" left leg and touch the toe on the ground but without shifting your weight. Bring your right hand up to guard your temple, turning to face diagonally outwards as it moves up. Your left hand floats down.

3 As you turn your waist to the left, your right hand follows and sweeps down; your left palm opens outwards.

4 As you turn your waist to the right, your right hand continues in a circle. Your left hand follows the move of your waist and faces down in front of your chest. As your waist returns to the centre, the right hand is level with the shoulder.

PLAY GUITAR. BRUSH LEFT KNEE AND PUSH

This posture is also known as "Strumming the Lute".

5 Take a shoulder-width step with your left foot, heel first. Move 70% of your weight into your left leg as your left hand brushes down across it. Meanwhile, your right hand follows a concave curve into the centre to finish by the mouth.

1 As all your weight sinks into your left leg, adjust the "empty" right foot by drawing it slightly nearer the left foot, toe first. Bring your weight into the right foot. Your left leg and arm float up simultaneously – imagine a thread connecting them.

2 Turn to the right, dropping your right hand down while your left hand follows the movement of your waist to the centre of your chest, palm facing down. As your waist returns to the front, your right hand comes to shoulder height.

STEP FORWARD, DEFLECT, INTERCEPT AND PUNCH

3 Take a shoulder-width step with your left foot, heel first. Move 70% of your weight into your left leg as your left hand brushes down across it. Your right hand follows a curve ending by your mouth.

1 Turn your waist 45° to the left and sink all your weight into your right foot. As the weight shifts back, lift the toes of your left foot and pivot 45° on the heel. Bring your hands down by your left leg.

2 Shift all your weight into your left leg. Form a loose fist with your right hand, but check that the fingers are not wrapped around the thumb. The right toes are behind the left heel.

3 Arc both of your hands and your right foot simultaneously towards the centre line, as your waist turns around to the right. The right foot now lands "empty", in line with the left instep. Check that your position is correct. Note that your left thumb should roughly be in line with your left eye.

4 Continue to turn your waist to the right, bringing the right fist palm upwards to rest on the right hip. You should now commence transferring all your weight on to your right foot. Your eyes should skim across the tops of your left fingers.

5 Place your left foot a shoulder width from the right foot. Shift 70% of your weight to your left leg and bring your right fist forward as if to punch, rotating it through a quarter turn in a corkscrew motion. Then bring your left arm across your body, with the palm facing your inner right elbow.

WITHDRAW AND PUSH. CROSSING HANDS

1 As you turn your waist to the left, your right arm follows your body to an angle of 45° and the fist opens up. Meanwhile, cup your left hand gracefully a couple of inches under your right elbow, as if supporting it.

2 Draw your right arm across your left palm as your weight sinks into your right foot, and your waist turns to the right.

3 Bring your waist back to the centre and turn both palms to face the front.

t'ai chi   51

4 Move your weight forward 70% on to your left leg. Your hands remain at shoulder width and shoulder height.

5 Turn your waist to the right and simultaneously sink all your weight into your left leg. Draw your hands in towards your chest in a softly inverted "V" shape, as if holding the top of a ball.

6 As your whole weight shifts into your right leg, turn your waist to the right. Your left toes turn with your waist and your right hand travels out both diagonally and upwards.

EMBRACE TIGER, RETURN TO MOUNTAIN

7 Sink all your weight back into your left leg. Your left hand now travels out diagonally. Though the position might seem slightly awkward and lopsided, it actually flows naturally into the final step.

8 Finally, bring your right foot shoulder-width away from and parallel to the left, but maintain your weight 70% in the left leg. Both hands circle down and up, stopping opposite your chest, palms facing the body. The wrists are touching, with the right wrist outside the left one. Hold this stance for a few seconds.

1 Keeping all your weight in your left leg, turn your waist to the right. Open your hands outwards. Step diagonally back with your right foot. Move your weight 70% on to your right foot. As your waist completes its turn, move your left hand so that the fingertips are in line with your left shoulder, palm facing forward.

ROLL BACK, PRESS AND PUSH: SINGLE WHIP

PUNCH UNDER ELBOW

2 As you turn your waist slightly to the right, allow your left hand to come across so that the fingertips point to your right elbow. Meanwhile, your right hand travels upwards so that the fingertips point heavenward.

1 Now repeat the sequence in "Roll Back, Press and Push". This time, perform this section from one diagonal corner to the other rather than from one side to the other. This picture shows your position at the end of the sequence.

1 Sink all your weight back on to your right foot. Turn your waist 45° to the left, lifting the left toes and letting your left foot and both arms pivot 45° to the left.

2 Lower your left foot, gradually shifting your weight forward into it. When all your weight is on your left foot, step forward with your right foot so that the heel is in line with your left instep.

3 Rotate your upper body 90° to the left. Your arms follow this waist movement, so that the hook (your right hand) is now out in front level with your right shoulder, and your left hand is level with your face at 90° to the front. Your weight is in your left leg.

4 Transfer all your weight to your right leg, turning your waist to the right and letting your left hand move down, then up, until the fingers are in line with your left shoulder. Your left arm and leg move around simultaneously. Rest your left heel on the ground without any weight.

STEP BACK TO REPULSE THE MONKEY

1 As you turn your waist further to the right, your right hand opens and moves down by your hip, then floats up to shoulder height. The palm of your left hand turns over to face down.

2 Step back with your left foot as your waist turns to the left. Your right hand travels forward, palm facing down, while your left hand travels down towards the left hip with the palm facing up.

3 The right toes also straighten as the waist turns. As you continue to turn to the left, your left hand floats up to shoulder height, while your right hand comes forward, palm facing down.

STEP BACK TO REPULSE THE MONKEY (RIGHT). DIAGONAL FLYING

1 Turn your waist to the right, step back with your right foot and let your left hand travel forward, palm down. Your right hand moves down to rest on your hip, palm up. Your left foot turns to face the front as the waist moves. Your right hand now comes up to shoulder height.

2 With your weight on your left foot, turn your waist to the left. Turn your right hand palm upwards as it travels round in front of your waist, while your left hand, palm downwards, comes in front of your chest. Your hands are now holding an imaginary ball in front of you.

3 Turn your waist 90° to the right, maintaining the position of your arms and hands in front of your chest, as if carrying the ball.

WAVING HANDS IN CLOUDS (RIGHT, LEFT, RIGHT)

4 Stepping with your right foot, turn a further 135° to the right, and then transfer 70% of your weight into the right foot. Your waist also turns to the right and your right hand moves with it, travelling to shoulder height, arm extended and facing diagonally upwards. Your left hand moves simultaneously to just outside your left thigh, palm facing down.

1 Bring all your weight on to your right foot. Turn your waist to the right and move your left hand across near your right hip. At the same time, your right hand turns palm downwards at shoulder height. Raise your left foot and move it forward until the left heel is now level and in line with the right.

2 As your waist turns to the front, move your right hand to face it and your left hand to face your chest. The right toes swivel round to face forwards so that your feet are now shoulder-width apart.

3 As your waist turns to the left, turn your palms towards each other, as if holding a large ball to the left of your body. All your weight is in your left leg and your right foot steps in to about half shoulder width.

4 Turn your waist back to the centre. Your hands again change position, the left hand descending to be opposite and facing your waist, and the right hand opposite and facing your chest.

5 Turn your waist to the right, your hands holding the imaginary ball, with the right hand uppermost, palm facing down, and the left hand below it, palm facing up. When all your weight is on your right foot, step back to shoulder-width apart.

WAVING HANDS IN CLOUDS (LEFT, RIGHT, LEFT). THE WHIP

1 Turn your waist back to the centre, bringing your right hand down to face your waist and your left hand up to face your chest. Repeat Steps 3, 4 and 5, then Steps 2 and 3 from "Waving Hands in Clouds, Right, Left, Right".

2 Turn your waist back to the centre and form a hook with your right hand, as it moves in level with your chest, directly above your left hand. It is located in front of your waist, palm upwards.

3 Step forward with your right foot. Turn your waist to the right, then to the left as you transfer your weight to your right foot, sending out the hook at 90° to the front of your body.

GOLDEN ROOSTER STANDS ON ONE LEG (LEFT). SQUATTING SINGLE WHIP

4 Continue turning your waist around towards the left, and then step with your left foot to about shoulder-width apart, with your left palm now facing your left shoulder.

5 Shift your weight 70% on to your left foot, turning away your left palm at shoulder height, and turning the right toes to 45°.

1 Sink all your weight into your left leg, turning your left hand over so that the palm faces upwards. Simultaneously turn out the right toes. This is a nicely balanced, elegant position.

2 Move your weight across into your right leg, bringing your left palm in towards your chest. The left toes turn 45° to the right.

3 Sink down into your right leg, keeping your back straight. Move your waist to the left, brush open your left knee with your left arm and turn your left toes out 90° to the left.

4 Transfer all your weight into your left leg. Open the right hand hook, lower the hand then bring it up in front of your chest. Raise your right leg as your weight shifts forward into your left leg, so that your right thigh becomes parallel with the ground. Bend your left knee.

GOLDEN ROOSTER STANDS ON ONE LEG (RIGHT). SEPARATE RIGHT FOOT

1 Place your right foot down and move all your weight on to it. As your weight sinks into your right leg, your right hand descends to rest on a cushion of air by your right thigh. Your left arm and left leg simultaneously move up to form a mirror image of the previous posture.

2 Step out with your "empty" left foot diagonally to the left, and form a ward-off position with your left arm horizontally positioned across your body, opposite your chest.

3 Shift all your weight into your left leg, bringing your right arm up to cross in front of your left arm, with the wrists touching. Bring your right toe to your left heel. Turn your wrists, maintaining skin contact as you do so, so that your left arm now crosses your right.

t'ai chi

SEPARATE LEFT FOOT, BRUSH LEFT KNEE AND PUSH

4 Then turn your hands away from your body, and open them out in a fan-like action. Your eyes should be level with the tips of your fingers.

5 Keep your left hand level with your left ear, palm facing away. Open out your right hand to the corner, below shoulder height, and simultaneously kick gently with your right leg, to knee height. You should be so balanced that you do not fall over.

1 Keeping all your weight in your left leg, turn to the left-hand corner, forming a ward-off position with your right arm.

2 Turn your waist to the right and step to the right with your right leg. As you transfer weight into it, bring your left hand up outside the right so that the wrists meet. The left toes come up to meet the right heel.

3 Open out your hands, the right hand this time remaining level with the head and the left hand travelling to below shoulder height. The left foot follows, kicking gently to the corner.

4 Turn your waist and left knee to the front again. Take a shoulder-width "empty" step with your left leg, toes pointing in the forward direction.

NEEDLES AT SEA BOTTOM

5 Brush your left hand across and above the front of your left leg, to just outside your left thigh. Your right hand curves in, fingertips forward, to finish with the fingers in line with your mouth.

1 Move all your weight into your left leg. Pick up your empty right foot and make a small adjustment step forward.

2 Place your right toes down, then bring your left hand across your body so that the left palm rests above your right wrist. At the same time, pick up your left leg and place the toes down.

IRON FAN PENETRATES BACK. TURN BODY, CHOP AND PUSH

3 Move your right arm forwards and diagonally downwards with your body, then vertically downwards. The arm remains in line with your right leg, and all your weight remains in your right leg.

1 Your weight remains in your right leg and both hands assume a ward-off position. Take a shoulder-width step with the left foot. Shift your weight 70% into your left leg and turn your hands outwards, the left hand by your chest, the right guarding your temple.

2 Turn your waist to the right and sink all your weight back into your right leg, bringing your left toes round. Bring your left hand up, turning the palm diagonally outwards to guard the temple. At the same time, form a loose fist with your right hand, palm facing downwards.

3 Sink all your weight back on to your left leg. As you transfer the weight back, the fist descends in front of your groin.

4 Step to shoulder width with your right foot. Your right arm pivots at the elbow and your left arm folds across so that the left hand faces the right inner elbow. All your weight remains on your left leg. You are nicely balanced as shown above.

5 Transfer your weight forward 70% into your right leg. Your left arm pushes forward, fingertips in line with your left shoulder, and your right fist descends to your right hip, palm upwards. The left toes are at 45°.

STEP FORWARD, DEFLECT DOWNWARDS, INTERCEPT AND PUNCH, KICK WITH HEEL

1 Sink all your weight into the left leg as your waist turns to the left. Bring the right toe to the left heel. The right hand comes across the body, and the palm faces down by the left hip. The left hand is below the right hand, palm up. Go to "Step Forward, Deflect, Intercept and Punch" and repeat Steps 3, 4 and 5.

2 Sink your weight into your left leg, turning your waist to the right. Cross your wrists, the right outside the left. Sink the weight back into your right leg. Your waist turns left and your left foot pivots on the heel 45° to the left. Shift all your weight forward into your left leg, turning your hands palms outwards.

3 Open your hands out gracefully like a fan, the right hand to below shoulder height, the left hand at head height, palms facing away. Your right foot now comes up from the ground, and the heel kicks diagonally away.

BRUSH RIGHT KNEE AND PUSH. BRUSH LEFT KNEE AND PUNCH DOWN

1 Place your "empty" right foot on the ground, toes forward. Your right hand curves down to rest on a cushion of air outside your right thigh. Your left hand curves forward to push to the centre, fingertips in line with your mouth.

2 Sink back into your left leg, turning your waist to the right, with the palm of your left hand facing towards your body in the Yang-style ward-off position.

3 Transfer your weight forward into your right foot, with your left palm turning so that it faces downwards.

WARD OFF RIGHT. ROLL BACK, PRESS AND PUSH. WHIP

4 Take a shoulder-width step with your left foot and bring 70% of your weight onto it. Your right hand forms a loose fist, which comes over your hip and punches down the centre. Your left hand brushes your left leg and rests by the left knee.

1 Sink back into your right leg. Your left hand now assumes a ward-off position, the fingertips of your right hand pointing towards the centre of the left palm. Your right palm faces downwards. Gaze steadily and confidently forwards.

2 Turn your body 45° to the left, pivoting neatly on the left heel. Shift all your weight forward into your left leg. Your left arm should remain in this position, while your right hand now presses smartly down.

FAIR LADY WEAVES SHUTTLES (RIGHT AND LEFT)

3 Step through at shoulder width with your "empty" right foot. As you transfer 70% of your weight into it, your right hand comes up into a ward-off position opposite your chest, with the left fingertips now pointing towards the right palm, left palm downwards. Repeat "Roll Back, Press and Push" and "Single Whip".

1 Transfer your weight to your right leg as you turn your waist to the right, and turn the "empty" left toes through 90°. Bring your left hand across your body and under your elbow. Open the hook of your right hand and lower the right arm, palm turning to face upwards.

2 Sink your weight back into your left leg, turn your waist further to the right and turn out your right foot so the heel is in line with the left instep.

3 Sink your weight into your right leg, drawing your left arm across your right palm, and step at shoulder width to the left corner with your left foot. As you shift your weight forward into your left leg, turn both palms outwards.

4 Transfer your weight into your right foot and turn your waist and left foot to the right as far as possible (135°). Turn your palms to face your body, the right palm by the left elbow.

5 Sink your weight back into your left leg and draw your left arm across your right palm.

FAIR LADY WEAVES SHUTTLES (RIGHT AND LEFT)

6 Turn a further 135° right, to the corner. Step to shoulder width with your right foot, and shift 70% of your weight into it, pushing towards the centre of your mouth with your left hand. Bring the right hand up to guard your forehead, palm facing diagonally.

1 Turn to the left, sinking all your weight into your left leg. Pick up your right foot and draw it in. Transfer all your weight to your right foot, then step to the left (45°) with your left foot. Turn your palms in and draw your right arm across the left palm, left arm in a ward-off position.

2 Your left hand then moves up and turns outwards by your head, while the fingers of your right hand come into the centre in line with your mouth. Now repeat the postures described in Steps 4, 5 and 6 of the previous exercise.

WARD OFF LEFT. WARD OFF RIGHT. ROLL BACK, PRESS AND PUSH. SINGLE WHIP

1 Sink your weight into your left leg as your waist turns to the left. Both arms come round with the movement of your waist, the left hand lower than the right. The right toes come round to the front.

2 Sink your weight into your right leg as your left hand presses down, palm facing downwards. Take a shoulder-width step with your left foot.

3 Transfer your weight 70% into your left foot. Your left hand comes up in front of your chest. Your right hand floats outside your right thigh. Repeat previous step.

SQUATTING SINGLE WHIP. STEP FORWARD FOR SEVEN STARS   RIDE TIGER

1 Repeat the postures described in Steps 1, 2 and 3 of "Golden Rooster Stands on One Leg (Left). Squatting Single Whip", ending by brushing open the left knee.

2 Transfer all your weight into your left leg. The right hand hook opens and the hand descends, then comes up in front of your neck, where it forms a loose fist. At the same time, your left hand rises up to form a loose fist, and connects at the wrist inside your right hand. Move your right toes forward to touch the ground without any weight whatsoever.

1 Keep your weight in your left leg and step back with your right foot, toes touching the ground first. Sink your weight into it and turn your waist to the right. The fists open and then move down by your right hip, with the wrists still connected.

2 Pick up your left leg as your waist turns right, then place your toes down as your waist turns back to the left. Your right hand comes round to the front, fingertips level with your right ear, and your left hand rests by your left thigh.

3 Pick up your left toes, turn your waist to the left corner and place the toes down empty of any weight. Your right palm faces your inner left elbow. Your left hand is at the height of your left shoulder, elbow relaxed.

4 Lift your left toes and swing your waist clockwise, pivoting on the ball of your right foot. Your arms swing to the right with the movement of your waist.

5 Drop your left foot and transfer all your weight into it straight away. Look closely at the photograph above to check how you should be standing.

6 When your arms and waist reach the front (the arms at shoulder height and shoulder width with the palms facing downwards), your right foot lifts up and circles clockwise.

7 After circling, your right leg comes to rest with the upper leg parallel to the ground and the foot comfortably relaxed. Your left leg is bent while the arms are still pointing ahead.

BEND BOW TO SHOOT TIGER. STEP FORWARD, DEFLECT DOWN, INTERCEPT AND PUNCH

1 Turn your waist to the right. Your arms follow your waist, dropping down parallel, and your right foot is placed facing the right corner.

2 As your waist turns to the right, shift the weight into your right leg and circle your arms round to the right. As your waist turns back to the left, raise your arms and circle round with the waist. Form loose fists. Bring the right hand up to the right of your forehead, knuckles facing the right eyebrow. The left hand is at shoulder height.

3 Sink your weight into your left leg and pick up your right foot, placing the toes by your left heel. Open the left fist as your arms move across your body following the waist movement.

WITHDRAW AND PUSH.
CROSSING HANDS. CONCLUSION.

4 Both hands and your right foot simultaneously arc in towards the centre line, as your waist turns to the right. The right foot lands "empty", completely in line with the left instep.

5 Continue to turn your waist, bringing the right fist palm upwards to rest on your right hip and shifting your weight to the right foot. Step through at shoulder width with your left foot. Shift 70% of your weight to the left and bring your right fist forward to punch in a corkscrew. Your left arm comes across your body.

1 Repeat the postures described in "Withdraw and Push. Crossing Hands". Ensure your weight is 70% in your left leg when crossing hands.

2 From crossing the hands, turn both palms down to face the ground as your body now rises up.

3 Bring all your weight into your left leg, turn your waist to the right and pivot on your left heel, turning the foot out to an angle of 45°.

4 Move all your weight into your right leg. Step in with your left foot so that the feet make a right angle. Bring half your weight to the left foot. Rest your arms and hands by your side with shoulders relaxed. You may now begin again.

yoga stretches

Have you ever watched a cat waking up? More often than not, it will give an exaggerated yawn, then arch its back until stretched to its limit, before loosely letting go and gracefully moving off on its way. Have you ever stopped to wonder why it makes these movements? The cat knows instinctively the value of stretching in maintaining flexibility and improving circulation to the muscles; you too can become stronger and more flexible with regular stretching exercises.

Most of us tend to hold in patterns of tension arising from everyday cares and worries, bad posture, lack of exercise and so on. These patterns make us feel stiff and unbending, and directly interfere with our movements. Inflexibility within our bodies can in turn affect mental flexibility, and we can become stuck in thought as well as in action. Regular stretching exercises not only free our bodies, allowing us to move easily, but can also help us to think and act without being so restricted. They are excellent improvers. In fact, by stretching muscles, ligaments and tendons, we make them much more efficient and stronger. The lengthening actions also help us to stand and walk taller, and even with added grace. The joints are better supported and are more able to go through their full range of movements, while the muscles are better nourished from the increased blood supply. The stretches give you that extra edge.

warm-up exercises

As any athlete will tell you, before starting to do any serious stretching or exercise, such as tennis, it is important that you first do some gentle warm-up exercises. They ensure that your muscles are nicely warmed and loosened, and will help to prevent any sudden strain or injury. The best thing is they only take a few minutes, and they can also be practised at any time if you are feeling stiff and need to loosen up.

SHRUGGING SHOULDERS

1 Stand upright with your feet slightly apart and your shoulders relaxed.

2 Lift your shoulders up as high as they will go, then let them fall down again. Stay relaxed and repeat a few times.

ARM CIRCLING

1 Wheel your arms around from the shoulders in slow, large circles.

2 Do this a few times going backwards, then repeat circling your arms forwards.

SQUATS

1 Stand with your feet slightly apart, hands on hips. Go slowly into a squat.

2 Slowly return to a standing position, then repeat. Your back should be upright.

LOOSE TWISTS

1 In a standing position with feet comfortably apart and knees relaxed, swing your arms loosely backwards and forwards around your body. Keep your head and body facing forward all the time, and keep your feet and pelvis still. Repeat a few times to loosen your arms and shoulders.

ARM STRETCHING

1 Stand with your arms straight out in front of you, at chest height. Take in a deep breath and exhale.

SIDEWAYS BEND

1 Stand with your feet at least shoulder-width apart and your arms hanging down at your sides. Bend down to one side, trying not to twist. Slowly return to the upright and then bend to the other side. Straighten up and now repeat.

SHAKE

1 Try to relax and let your whole body go completely floppy. Shake your limbs to release any tension. Continue for as long as you feel comfortable. If you prefer, shake each limb in sequence, starting with your right arm.

CAT STRETCH

1 Kneel on all fours, with your hands and knees shoulder-width apart. As you start to inhale, bring your head forward and slightly hollow your back.

2 Now breathe out and, as you do so, arch the back upwards like a cat, allowing your head to drop down. Repeat a few times.

therapeutic movements

One of the best things about stretches is that you can do some simple, straightforward exercises anywhere, at any time: at home, in the office, standing in a queue or even sitting in the car; there are no restrictions. However, in order to get the most benefit from regular stretching, and particularly from doing yoga practice, it is important to create a quiet, comfortable space and to give yourself plenty of time to do the movements without any pressure or interruptions from the telephone or colleagues. In fact, making this space is in itself a relaxing, unwinding step, and will enhance the effectiveness of the actual exercises.

Ideally, make an area that feels quiet and calming to you, perhaps with softer lighting if it is needed, maybe with a thick, soft mat for the floor-based stretches. If you have any back discomfort, or just need extra support when lying down, then a couple of cushions may be extremely useful. It is helpful to wear loose fitting, airy clothing so that you can move freely and easily. If the weather permits try to let in some fresh air, but do not risk getting cold. These exercises are not intended to work up a good sweat or strain the heart, but to make you feel altogether less stiff and tense, and generally much more flexible. They are great for loosening you up, releasing tensions, improving circulation, toning the body, and generally making you feel much freer and more confident with your own body. They can really perk you up. After each exercise you will also need time to relax quietly, before you plunge back into everyday life.

If you find them an enormous benefit and become inspired, and want to try out more exercises, then do find a good, local class. Yoga exercises are generally best learnt in such a class, with a skilled, experienced teacher for maximum benefit. Alternatively you could create your own class at home, inviting a yoga teacher, friends and family on a regular basis.

tension and backache relievers

In the great majority of cases back trouble is the result of chronic tensions which can build up around the spine. Tired, tight muscles are also much more prone to strain or injury. The stretches that are shown here are intended to aid flexibility of the spine, and to make you feel much more supple, but if you already suffer from back pain or an injury then you must seek professional advice.

COBRA

1 Lie on your front, with your arms bent and your hands under your shoulders.

2 Slowly lift your head and push down on your arms to help raise your trunk.

3 If you can, tilt your head backwards and stretch up and back, then relax.

SIMPLE TWIST

1 Sit on the floor with your legs stetched straight out in front of you.

2 Bend one leg and place the foot on the floor across the other knee.

3 Place your opposite arm in front of your bent leg and twist to look over your shoulder.

FULL TWIST

1 Bend one leg so that the foot rests on the inner thigh of the other leg.

2 Bring this leg over the first one, then grasp your foot with the other arm.

3 Twist as far around as you can, hold, then relax. Swap over your legs. Repeat.

TRIANGLE

1 Stand with your feet shoulder-width apart and your arms straight out to the sides. This should be a well-balanced, easily held position. Your head should feel like a ball balancing on your neck. Stare straight ahead.

2 Bend down to one side without twisting your body, letting the opposite arm rise in the air. If you find this awkward or uncomfortable, do not strain yourself. The object is to loosen the body, not injure it.

3 Stretch the raised arm, look up and hold. Slowly straighten and repeat on the other side. If you can, repeat several times, but be careful to move slowly into position to avoid a strain.

BENDING TWIST

1 Stand with your feet shoulder-width apart and your arms straight out to the sides. Bending forward, try to touch your foot, or the floor in front of it if you can, with your opposite hand. Slowly uncurl and return to the starting position. Repeat on the other side.

SLOUCH STRESS

1 Sit on a tall stool so that your feet are just off the floor. With your hands behind your back, slouch so that your back is rounded, with your head now lowered down towards your chest.

2 Flex one foot, and lift the leg to straighten it if possible. Release the leg, relax, then repeat a few times. Repeat with the other leg. Note that the object is to build up a slow pace, not to go fast.

soothing and removing tension

Many of us suffer at some time from tension headaches and know that they begin with a gradual feeling of pressure in the head or neck, or a taut sensation in the facial muscles. Once you are aware of such tension, tackle it immediately. A few simple stretches can help to relieve these muscular spasms and prevent them leading to a severe headache. They can be done almost anywhere.

SIDEWAYS NECK STRETCH

1 Slowly stretch your head down to one side, feeling the pull in the neck muscles. Return the head to the upright position and repeat on the other side.

2 To make this stretch of the neck muscles more effective, use your hands to give extra leverage. Place one hand under your chin and the other on top of your head; repeat the other side.

HEAD TO CHEST

1 Lower your head towards your chest, feeling the pull on the back of the neck. Hold at your furthest stretch before slowly raising the head again. Repeat two or three times.

LION POSTURE

1 To stretch the facial muscles and release tension, open your mouth as wide as possible and push out your tongue. At the same time, open your eyes into as wide a stare as you can manage. Repeat a couple of times.

SEMICIRCLE ROTATION

1 Turn the head to one side, then steadily rotate it in a semicircular movement, letting the chin drop down across the chest.

2 Dropping the head backwards compresses the neck, so it is best not to make this a full circle rotation. Repeat, going back in the opposite direction.

posture enhancers

One of the great benefits of an exercise system such as yoga is the fact that it gradually and increasingly gives you considerable grace and poise. In addition it will make a huge difference to your overall posture. If it was previously a bit lax, and you ended up slouching, you will really notice the difference. In fact, learning to hold yourself properly can help you to look and feel much younger, and reduce muscle strain.

1 Stand with feet slightly apart and arms raised in front. Slowly twist to one side. Repeat on the other side.

2 Stand with your feet apart, and hold your arms out. Bend over, sliding one hand down the inside of the same leg.

3 Reach as far as is comfortable, then slowly return to the upright and repeat on the other side.

4 For the tree routine, stand on one leg and bend the other knee, as shown.

5 Either place your palms together above your head, or raise the hands.

6 For the arm and leg stance, stand on one leg and hold the other foot behind.

tired and aching leg revivers

Most of us spend too long each day with our legs stuck in fixed positions, and stiffness of the lower limbs from inactivity or tension can make you feel quite tired. Legs benefit from being stretched, keeping them toned and supple. These exercises prevent the legs, thighs and lower back from getting too tense. Since some of these positions are quite difficult, do beware of straining yourself.

ALTERNATE LEG PULLS

1 Sit on the floor, with one leg out straight and the other bent so that the foot rests on the inner thigh of your extended leg. Do it with care.

2 Lean forward and clasp the straight leg as far down as is comfortable; pull your chest down a little further and hold for a moment. Change legs and repeat.

FULL LEG PULLS

1 The previous stretch can be extended by starting with both legs straight out in front of you. Repeat as described.

SIDE LEG RAISE

2 Lean forward and hold the legs with both hands; pull yourself down a little further and hold for a moment. If this is difficult, bend the legs slightly.

1 Lie on your side with your legs and body in a straight line. Support your head with one hand and place your free hand on the floor for balance.

2 Without twisting your hips, steadily raise the upper leg as far as is comfortable. Hold, then lower slowly. Repeat with the other leg.

CAT STRETCH

1 Kneel on all fours with your hands and knees shoulder-width apart. Raise your head and look straight ahead.

2 Breathe in, and as you exhale lift and arch your back. Hold for a moment before relaxing back into the original position. Inhale, then repeat.

BACK PUSH-UP

1 Lie on your back with your knees bent and your feet on the floor, hip-width apart. Now place your hands on the floor by your shoulders.

2 Push up with your hands and feet, arching your back at the same time. Hold for a moment, then lower your body back to the floor. Do not strain yourself with this movement – it works on lots of muscles at the same time.

SIT UP/LIE DOWN

1 Sit on the floor with both legs straight out in front of you. Your torso should be at right angles to your legs, with your eyes looking forward.

2 Slowly lower your back to the floor, then start to bend the legs and raise them off the floor.

3 As you raise the legs, slowly start to straighten them until they are as close to the vertical as you can manage. Again, take care not to strain yourself.

4 Keeping the legs straight, slowly lower them to the floor.

5 Continue the movement by sitting up and clasping your legs with your hands to bend forwards. Slowly return to the original sitting position.

abdominal tension relievers

We tend to hold and lock up too much tension in our abdomen, especially if we are the kind of people who always bottle up our feelings. Even simple muscular tension can leave us feeling stiff and rather uncomfortable, and much less flexible around the waist. Consequently exercises aimed at reducing stiffness and increasing flexibility in the abdominal region are extremely useful.

LOTUS

1 For the full lotus, the first leg should be bent with the foot on top of the other thigh, and the second leg bent so that the foot goes over the other leg on to the opposite thigh. Hold if possible.

2 For an easier version bend one leg and rest the foot on the inner thigh of the other leg. Bend the second leg and place the foot on top of the opposite thigh. Keep the spine upright.

ABDOMINAL MOVEMENTS

1 Either sit cross-legged or kneel, and place your hands on your waist or thighs. Breathe out completely.

2 Without inhaling, pull in your abdomen as far as you can, then "snap" it in and out up to five times before taking a breath. Relax for a few moments, breathing freely, before repeating.

LEG OVER

1 Lie on your back, with your legs out straight. Raise one leg as close to the vertical as is comfortable, then move it across the body, keeping your hips in contact with the floor.

2 Push the leg as far over as possible, then slowly return to the original position. Repeat with the other leg.

yoga stretches

LYING TWISTS

1 Lie on your back, hands behind your head and legs together, knees bent.

2 Twist the legs from side to side, keeping the back and hips on the floor.

SIDE BENDS

1 Stand with feet apart and hands on hips. Bend down to one side.

ROLL TWIST

2 Slowly return to the upright position and bend to the other side. Repeat.

1 Keeping the legs and hips still, roll your upper body around in a clockwise circle.

2 Move slowly and carefully, and bend only as far as is comfortable.

SIT UP/LIE DOWN

1 Sit on the floor with both legs straight out in front of you.

2 Slowly lie back, then start to bend the legs and raise them off the floor.

3 Sit up, bend forwards, clasp your legs and slowly return to the sitting position.

office tensions and stiff muscles

For people who spend their working day sitting at a desk it is very easy to get stiff, aching muscles. Badly designed chairs do not help, and as you get tired, so posture suffers and you can end up getting round-shouldered. It is therefore absolutely essential that every now and again you get up and walk around, relax your body, and try some of these excellent loosening-up exercises.

SEATED CAT STRETCH

1 Pull the chair back from the desk slightly to give yourself more room, then bend forward and clasp your ankles.

2 Carefully arch your back to stretch, then relax back and repeat.

CALF STRETCH

1 Sit fairly upright, then lift and straighten each leg alternately. Repeat a few times.

2 Flex the foot to stretch the calf muscle. Repeat a few times.

NECK TWISTS

1 Turn your head to one side, feeling the extension in the neck muscles.

2 Repeat, turning the head from side to side. Do both steps quite slowly.

ARM AND CHEST STRETCH

I Sitting upright, link your hands together, palms away from your body, and push your arms straight out in front of you. Hold for a couple of seconds, relax and then repeat.

ARM AND BACK STRETCH

I Link your hands together behind your back, over the top of the chair, and lift your arms slightly. Do not strain yourself. Push away from your body, hold, then repeat the exercise.

FOREARM STRETCH

I Hold your arms straight out to the sides and stretch them. Alternately flex and extend your hands. Feel the pull on the upper and lower sides of your forearms as you do so.

BACK/SHOULDER STRETCH

I Stretch your arms up in the air over your head. As you breathe in, arch your back ever so slightly. Relax with the exhalation and repeat the exercise a couple of times.

POSTURE CLASP

I Put one arm behind your back and bend it up, with the hand reaching the other shoulder. With your other arm raised and bent down over your shoulder, try to clasp your fingers.

SHOULDER RELEASE

I Link your fingers together and stretch your arms high above your head. Repeat several times.

meditation

Meditation has been in use from the beginning of time: people have always sought inner quiet and physical relaxation, whether for reasons connected with the spirit, self-realization or health. You do not have to be a physical contortionist to achieve and enjoy the benefits of meditation at both physical and mental levels.

What, then, is meditation? It has been described as just sitting and relaxing. Many people find that their lives are so full of the demands of work, family, friends and organized leisure pursuits that they have no time to "stand and stare". Many are so caught up in planning and working towards the future that they take little pleasure from the here and now. In their bustle to "get on" they miss out on the simple pleasures of life. But beauty and joy are there to be seen and experienced, even in industrial cities.

The benefits of meditation come from regular use. If you are under stress, you may find that meditating twice daily will be effective in restoring composure. Make a time and space you can call your own, and use breathing and relaxation exercises to ease yourself into the meditative state. The more you practise meditation the less time you will need to spend on these, but they remain useful in calming and preparing you. Allow at least 10 minutes, ideally 20, for meditation in each session.

the benefits of meditation

Human beings were never designed to cope with the high-pressure demands of life in the 21st century; life when you are constantly in demand, having to make vital decisions at breakneck speed right through the day, and even during the night. You might say it cannot be done, but it can, with help. Knowing how as well as when to switch off makes all the difference, and even scientists now agree.

PSYCHO-PHYSICAL LINKS

A period of meditation can often lead to a feeling of being refreshed, with a more positive attitude and a general feeling of well-being. Things that had been bothering you may now be seen in a new and more helpful way. You gain a different, wider perspective on things and feel very much more in control.

These beneficial reactions have been well known for years, but only in recent times has anyone found a physiological explanation. Detailed, extensive knowledge of brain scans and even brain wave patterns has given extraordinary new information about what is commonly called the "alpha state".

Mind and body work together in meditation to promote health and well-being in the whole person.

Endorphin Release

When we are truly relaxed, both mentally and physically, there are changes in the brain wave pattern until it is predominantly located and fixed within the alpha state. Within this particular state the brain triggers chemicals known as endorphins. It is in fact this chemical trigger that has the benefits that are experienced as a feeling of well-being. Indeed, endorphins have frequently been called "nature's very own special opiates". Meditation is one of the easiest ways to achieve this, and these good feelings can easily linger for some time after the meditation has ended, the length of time varying considerably. There is also a real physical benefit, as these endorphins boost and recharge the immune system, helping you to fight off all kinds of infections.

Meditation and Work

The tensions of modern working practices often mean that people are so bound up in meeting all the vigorous demands placed upon them that they maintain a high level of mental and physical activity right through the day. This frequently means that they are not only cutting off their extremely important emotional responses and their enjoyment of the simple things in life, but they are also pushing their physical and mental health right to the very limit. Much has now been written about the management of stress, and the significant need for periods of mental and physical relaxation during the working day.

The 20-minute Rule

One writer, Ernest Rossi, has formulated the 20-minute rule which is based on the theory of ultradian rhythms. Ultradian rhythms are biorhythms that the body works through during each day – a little like hyperbolic curves of energy which repeat every 90 to 120 minutes. Naturally, it would be best to work only at peak performance times, but this is just not possible. However, timing work breaks to coincide with the mind/body slow-down pattern every 90 minutes does ensure maximum productivity and restricts the potential build-up of stress.

Rossi suggested the pattern of working for 90 minutes and then taking a brief 20-minute break. He himself usually lies down and meditates during this period because it is the best form of total mental and physical relaxation, and is good preparation for returning to optimum mental processing.

It is important that these breaks take place every 90 minutes or so, and in such a way as to completely change the mind/body state. Ideally, you should stop all work activity and experience a change of physical status (standing rather than sitting, looking into the distance rather than close up, for example) and mental focus. A 20-minute meditation is ideal and the benefits will be felt immediately. On returning to work after the 20 minutes, you will see things afresh and deal with them more efficiently, as you are ready to climb to peak performance on the biorhythmic curve. The feeling of well-being lasts into the next 90-minute period.

To be at your best for meetings ensure you take regular breaks.

gaining the meditative state

Many religious groups, as well as adherents of Transcendental Meditation, use a sound, or "mantra", to help with meditation. The constant repetition of a phrase, word or sound ("aum" is commonly used in Hinduism) creates the alpha state by an almost hypnotic focus of attention upon that particular sound. In fact chants repeated again and again can lead to its members reaching a "high".

Sound

An effortless sound, repeated with the natural regular rhythm of breathing, can have the same soothing, liberating effect as the constant natural sound of running water, rustling leaves or a beating heart. The single sound, or mantra as it is known, is used to blot out the "chatter" of intrusive thoughts, allowing the mind to find deep repose. Speaking or chanting a mantra as a flowing stream of endless sound is a very old method of heightening a person's awareness by concentrating the senses. The simple gentle sound "om", or "aum", is sometimes known as the first mantra, which is literally an instrument of thought. The curving Sanskrit (the ancient language of Hindus in India) symbol for this primordial word represents the various states of consciousness: waking, dreaming, deep sleep and the transcendental state.

However, the actual sound need not be a special word or incantation; something simple and meaningful will be as effective. The sound of the word "calm" spoken or thought with each exhalation can be very effective, especially while imagining tension leaving your body. Any word that appeals to you will do.

Make sure that you are sitting quite comfortably and then start breathing in the colour of your choice.

Repeating a mantra takes you into a world of peace and harmony.

Touch

You can use your sense of touch in a lulling, soothing way to induce a state of meditation at times of stress. Young children do this when they adopt a satisfyingly smooth ribbon or piece of fabric to hold and manipulate when they are feeling tense. The same technique is seen all over the Middle East, where strings of worry beads are rhythmically passed through the fingers at difficult moments to focus the mind and calm anxiety. Their uniform size, gentle round shapes, smooth surfaces and rhythmic, orderly clicking as they are passed along their string all assist the meditative state. Use one or two smooth, rounded stones in the same way, passing them slowly from hand to hand.

Colours

Some colours are associated with relaxation and can be a helpful way to clear the mind of tension and allow meditation to start. Sit with your eyes closed, and be aware of the colour that comes into your mind: it may be any colour of the rainbow – red or purple are common. Then slowly and gradually allow that colour to change to a blue or green colour, allowing it to fill the whole of your mind's eye and replacing all other colours. The colour pink is also recommended by colour therapists and this may prove helpful. You will find a feeling of relaxation growing as the new colour builds in your mind, and when the relaxed colour is complete, you will experience feelings of inner peace.

Establish a comfortable rhythm of breathing and then focus on it until your mind is completely still, relaxed and clear. Colours are associated with all kinds of qualities, so choose the best for your own particular moods and needs. Red: vitality, energy, strength and willpower (complementary colour turquoise). Orange: happiness and laughter (complementary colour blue). Yellow: intellect and objectivity (complementary colour violet). Green: cleansing and harmony (complementary colour magenta). Turquoise: boosts and strengthens the immune system, counteracts disease (complementary colour red). Blue: peace and relaxation, restful sleep (complementary colour orange). Violet: beauty, dignity, assured self-respect (complementary colour yellow). Magenta: the liberating release of all obsessional thoughts and memories (complementary colour green).

how to use meditation

The key to using meditation lies in recognizing that you actually need it. Once you get into the whirlpool of work and stress, they can both all too easily become an integral part of your lifestyle. In fact, they can be such a formidable cornerstone that you cannot imagine what life could possibly be like without them. But once you stand back and see clearly and exactly what is happening to you, what your life has become, then suddenly you see you actually need a way out. One of the best ways involves deep meditation.

Meditation needs to be done like regular exercise. In fact you might say you are exercising the ways in which you relax. The very first step involves switching off, like switching off a light in a room, and concentrating on what could be called the "Inner Other", that is to say the marvellous, relaxed, empty inner spaces inside your head and body. This stage, put crudely, means sweeping out all the noise and mayhem and chaos of everyday life and getting ready to enter another world.

The second stage involves being carried along what one expert teacher calls "a moving but going nowhere sound that coils round and even through itself in a perpetual state of being". Perhaps the best way of evaluating it is by hearing what people have to say after meditation. "As good as a holiday" or "like a wonderful deep refreshing sleep" is what most people say. If you are to get its full, continuous benefits then you really must make sure that meditation is something that you do regularly every day, at certain times, because like almost all forms of exercise the more often you do it, the better you are at it; the quicker you can switch off and tune in, and enter that fantastic deep state of total energizing, refreshing relaxation.

You must use meditation with care though. It is not like switching on and off a tap. It needs to be respected. Few people who meditate try, even if they could, to describe its ultimate power. That would be like divulging a wonderful private secret; to have it is quite enough.

simple meditation techniques

If you want to learn to meditate seriously, you would do well to find an experienced teacher to guide you. However, there are many simple techniques that you can practise alone, often with quite powerful effects. Try the ones described here, and see which you feel in tune with. The more you practise, the easier it will become to reach a deep meditative state.

Introduce a child to meditation by using the Numbers Game.

THE NUMBERS GAME

This is a very simple form of meditation using a blackboard, real or imaginary. It is a good "game" to use with children (or adults), giving them a taste of meditation, and they really enjoy it. It is described here as if you are leading a group, but it can be easily used on one person, and provides an excellent way to clear the mind through concentration, imagination and patterns: all wonderful ways of gaining a real experience of deep meditation.

What you must do is this …

1 Get the children to sit or lie comfortably. Once they have found a really comfortable position ask them to remember it.
2 With chalk on the blackboard, draw a diagram of numbers, making sure that there are no mathematical links, like this:

```
3  1  5
8  6  9
4  7  2
```

3 Give the children one minute to memorize this sequence.
4 Ask them to return to their relaxed position, eyes closed, and concentrate on the numbers alone.
5 Rub out the numbers, telling them to do the same in their minds. Do this slowly saying "That leaves just four numbers", etc.
6 Then rub out the last number, saying "Now concentrate on what is left" … Let them remain in silence until you notice a restlessness – this is often three or more minutes.
7 Wake them gently with an instruction to "Sit up". Ask them what the last number was and for their reactions.

THE HAVEN

Once you have managed to achieve complete physical relaxation and calm, gradually allow your mind to enter a place, whether real or imaginary, that is quite special to you. Now you can allow your mind to drift … drift to a pleasant, peaceful place. A place that you know and where you always feel able to relax … completely. A safe … secure … place … where no one … and nothing can ever bother you.

It may be a place you have visited on holiday, a beach or a place in the countryside. Or it may be a room … a room you have had … a room you do have … or a room you would like to have … an imaginary place. But it is a place where you can always feel able to let go … completely … a haven, a haven of tranquillity, unique and special to you.

In order to help you imagine this place … notice first the light: is it bright, natural or dim … is there any particular source of light … natural or man-made? Notice also the temperature level … hot, warm or cool … and any particular source of heat. Be aware of the colours that surround you … shapes … and textures … the familiar objects that make that place special. Begin to see it in all its detail. You can just be there … whether sitting, lying or reclining, enjoying the sounds … the smells … the atmosphere … with nobody wanting anything, nobody needing anything and no one demanding anything from you. Relax.

Everyone has their own haven, a quiet magical place like this.

Try to imagine your perfect country house.

A GUIDED VISIT TO A COUNTRY HOUSE

Imagine that you are visiting a beautiful country house … a really beautiful old country house or a stately home with magnificent sweeping lawns on a warm, sunny, summer's afternoon. You are standing on the staircase that leads into the entrance hall, one of those wide ceremonial types of staircase. And as you look down across the entrance hall you can just glimpse, through the open doors opposite, a gravel drive, and the sunlight on the gravel. It is a beautiful, sunny, summer's afternoon and there is no one around to trouble or bother you as you stand alone on that staircase …

Now you are moving down the last ten steps to the hallway, relaxing more and more with each step down.

10 Taking one step down, relaxing and letting go …
9 Taking another step down, feeling at ease …
8 Becoming more relaxed, letting go even more …
7 Just drifting deeper … and deeper … everything is getting darker and darker, and even deeper down still …
6 Becoming calmer … and calmer … even calmer still …
5 Continuing to relax, continuing to let go and feeling good …
4 Relaxing even more … letting go even more …
3 Sinking deeper … drifting even further into this welcoming, relaxed state …
2 Enjoying those good feelings, all those feelings of inner peace and relaxation …
1 Nearly all the way down now, feeling very good … beautifully relaxed … and **0**.

You are wandering across that hallway now, towards the open doors and the gardens beyond, soaking up the atmosphere of peace and permanence in that lovely old building. You wander out through the doors and down the stone steps outside … and find yourself standing on the gravel drive outside, a wide gravel drive that leads down to the entrance gates.

As you stand there you notice the lush green lawns, so flat and well-clipped … and there are shrubs and trees, different shades of green and brown against a clear, blue sky … and you can feel the warmth of the sun on your head and shoulders as you enjoy this beautiful summer's afternoon in this lovely old garden … There are flowerbeds with their splashes of colour so carefully arranged and neatly tended. And there's no one else about … nobody needing anything, nobody wanting anything and nobody expecting anything from you, so you can enjoy the peace and serenity and solitude of this afternoon in this beautiful garden that's been so well looked after for so many, many years.

A little way down on the right-hand side of the driveway, you notice an ornamental fish pond. So you decide to wander down and have a look at those fish. Sometimes they seem almost to disappear behind the weed and shadows, but always they reappear, with their scales catching the sunlight, red, gold, silver or black. And as you watch those fish your mind becomes even more deeply relaxed …

THE WELL

This continues from the previous visualization of the beautiful country house and is intended to take you to even deeper levels of meditation.

… As you watch those fish you notice that the centre of the pond is very deep. It could be the top of a disused well. You take from your pocket a silver-coloured coin, and toss that coin so that it lands over the centre of the pond, and then you watch as it swings down through the water. The ripples drift to the edges of the pond, but you just watch that coin as it sinks deeper and deeper through that clear water, sometimes it seems to disappear as it turns on edge, at other times a face of the coin catches the sunlight and it flashes through the water … sinking, drifting deeper and deeper, twisting and turning as it makes its way down … Finally it rests at the bottom lying on a cushion of soft brown mud, a silver coin in that still, clean water on its own cushion of mud … And you feel as still as that coin, as still and cool and motionless as that water, enjoying that feeling of inner peace and stillness.

Watch the ripples as the coin lands in the very centre of the pond. Look even more closely as it tumbles down through the water …

personal development

Affirmations are a deceptively simple device that can be used by anyone and they are remarkably effective. Try to use this method while in the meditative state, having planned and memorized the affirmations involved. These powerful, positive phrases will improve communication with all parts of your mind. All you need is a simple phrase summing up how you want to be.

THE POWER OF WORDS
To make affirmations effective, they should
- be made in the present tense
- be positively phrased
- have an emotional reward.

Now contrast the power of such phrases with what happens if you are asked not to do or think of something. The words "no", "not", "never" and so on generally have the opposite effect to that intended, and why? Yours is the most influential voice in your life because you believe it. It comes live, straight out of the personality and intellect, and is fuelled by your dreams and language. The power you have over yourself is extraordinary. That is precisely why you must be careful to avoid any negative or demeaning statements you regularly make about yourself, either to others or to yourself – "I am shy", "I lack confidence", "I cannot", "I get nervous when" and so on – they are self-limiting beliefs that you are reinforcing each time they slip into your conversation or mind. You become what you say.

The point about affirmations is that instead of running yourself down, albeit in a subtle, insidious way, you actually start building yourself up. You start creating the inner psychological scaffolding to support the new you. Such affirmations are best used while in a wonderful state of meditation.

Thinking through what you want to be is the big key to success.

IMPROVED SELF-WORTH
We all have attributes and qualities in which we can take pride and pleasure. This exercise is about emphasizing these positive aspects to allay the doubts that only serve to limit our potential.
- I like my [physical attribute].
- I am proud of my [attitude or achievement].
- I love meeting people – they are fascinating.
- My contribution is valuable to [name person].
- I am lovable and can give love.
- Others appreciate my [opinions, assistance, a personal quality].
- I enjoy being a unique combination of mind and body.

Now imagine yourself speaking to colleagues, boss, employees or friends ... See yourself behaving and looking confident, standing and looking a confident person ... Notice how you stand ... your facial expression ... hear the way that you speak ... slowly, calmly, quietly, clearly and with confidence. You are communicating your needs ... ideas ... opinions in a positive way. Notice how your words flow easily, and how others are listening attentively to you ... valuing what you have to say. Now "climb aboard" ... be there – know how it feels to stand like that ... to speak like that ... and to have that positive reception from others. Get in touch with the stance ... expression ... and feelings ... and know that you can use these any time in the future to gain those same feelings or that inner strength in everything you do. See yourself in different situations: at home, in a social setting, in all the parts of your life, confident and assured, going from strength to strength.

The difference affirmations can make is extraordinary. From shy and introverted to open, confident and winning.

VISUALIZATION

In the same way that you can utilize your voice, so, perhaps more powerfully, you can use your imagination. The imagination can stimulate emotions, and they can register new attitudes in the mind. It can be a direct communication with the deeper levels of the mind, providing a powerful influence for improvements in your attitudes, behaviour patterns and overall confidence.

Visualization requires that you imagine yourself in a situation, behaving, reacting and looking as you would wish to do at an interview, an important meeting, a social gathering, a one-to-one situation, or perhaps a sporting event. Imagine what that will mean for you, your reactions, the reactions of those around you and, importantly, feel all the good feelings that will be there when this happens in reality.

It is like playing a video of the event, on that screen on the inside of the forehead, the mind's eye, from the beginning of the situation through to the perfect outcome. Should any doubts or negative images creep into your "video", push them away and replace them with positive ones. Keep this realistic, and base it upon real information from your past.

If you want to be No. 1, then take time to concentrate on seeing yourself as the best. Give yourself the power to come out top.

CONFIDENCE IN FUTURE SITUATIONS

The meditative state, affirmations and visualization can be a valuable rehearsal and preparation for a future event. Athletes and other sportsmen have proved that it actually does work. We can all use these extraordinary techniques to achieve our own optimum performance during any situation. Now consider the following phrases, and how they relate to you …

- I am quietly confident in meetings.
- I speak slowly, quietly and confidently so that others listen.
- My contribution is wanted and valued by others.
- I enjoy meetings, as they bring forth new ideas and help to renew my enthusiasm.

Imagine an important meeting that is about to happen, and see yourself there, filling in all the details that you know, and the people too; imagine yourself there looking confident and relaxed, concentrating on what is happening. Be aware of the acute interest you are giving to what is happening with complete, concentrated attention, and then imagine yourself speaking, to give information or to ask a question: hear yourself speaking quietly, slowly and calmly …

Notice people listening to what you are saying; they wish you well and support you, as you are expressing your viewpoint or raising a question they may well have wanted to ask, too. Notice how you are sitting or standing, how you lean slightly forward when speaking, that expression of calm confidence on your face. When this is clear in your mind, just like a film playing in your mind's eye, play it back and forth. When you are feeling comfortable with it, get into that imaginary you, "climb aboard" and be there in your mind, seeing things from that perspective, hearing things from that point in the meeting. As you speak, get in touch with those calm feelings, and the attitudes that allow you to feel calm, in control, and quietly confident … It is like a rehearsal; the more you manage to rehearse the better the final performance will be. You will acquire the right attitudes, stance and tone of voice, so that when you are in that situation all of these will be available to you, and it will be just as you imagined, as if you had done it all, successfully, before.

In short, what this technique does is take you step by step through a rehearsal. Imagine every possible scenario, and how you will deal with it. That is the key to a successful outcome.

The preparation was worth it; you went into a meeting knowing you could do it, and that is exactly what happened.

enjoyment and achievement

The mind and the body are so completely interlinked that if we keep physically fit we are also mentally alert. The one boosts the other, but it also works the other way around. If we really utilize our mental capacities we can affect and improve our physical health and performance. So it is up to you to make sure that these twin forces keep functioning at full power. Do not let either slip.

A well-tuned lively body keeps you feeling well and alert.

THE BODY/MIND LINK

Regularly say to yourself …
- I feel safe, happy and content in the knowledge that my body is constantly renewing itself. It is alive and well.
- It feels marvellous to know that every damaged cell is replaced by a healthy one.
- My immune system is strong and fights off any infections easily.
- My mind and my body are working in harmony to keep me healthy, well and alert.

Now, imagine yourself lying or sitting comfortably. As you see yourself there you notice a healing glow of coloured light surrounding your body, but not touching it. Let that colour become stronger, until it has a very clear pure colour, which is the colour of healing for you.

Now, as you watch, that healing, coloured light begins to flow into the top of your head. You can see it slowly draining into all parts of the head, face, ears, and starts its journey down through the neck and shoulders, into the tops of the arms … It continues to flow down through the arms and the chest area, that healing, coloured light, penetrating all the muscles and organs … even as you watch you can also feel a healing warmth coming into your body … NOW … as it flows down into the stomach area, the back, right the way down to the base of the spine. Then you can allow the light to disperse again and gradually return to your normal wakeful state, knowing that in those areas that need it, the healing process will continue.

STRESS REDUCTION

Stress is a factor in everyone's life and can even be a major motivator in some circumstances. Meditation can be a great help in coping with it, and combined with visualization, it can change your whole response to stressful demands. Keep saying …
- I enjoy solving problems.
- I work well under pressure.
- I am a calm, methodical and efficient worker.
- I love that feeling of having achieved so much in a day.
- I enjoy being calm when others around me are not.

Imagine yourself in a situation that has in the past caused stress. Picture the situation, and the other people involved … See yourself there … and notice a slight shimmer of light between yourself and those other people … a sort of bubble around you … a protective bubble that reflects any negative feelings back to them … leaving you able to get on with your tasks … your life, with an inner strength and calmness that surprises even you. A protective, invisible bubble surrounds you at all times. It will only allow those feelings that are positive and helpful to you to pass through for you to enjoy and build upon. Others may catch stress from each other … negativity, too, can be infectious … but you are protected … you continue to keep things in perspective … and to deal with things calmly and methodically. You are able to see the way forward clearly … solve problems … find ways around difficulties … by using your own inner resources and strengths, born of experience. In you alone lies the secret of success. You can and you will succeed.

Imagine yourself leading a healthy lifestyle and it will happen.

LIVING NOW

Although we cannot change the past, we can learn from it and build up a range of skills and useful insights from it. The future is that unknown world of possibilities and opportunities before us – but all that we can truly have any effect upon is the present. Keep saying to yourself …
- I have learned a great deal from the past.
- The future is an exciting range of opportunities.
- I enjoy laying good foundations NOW on which to build a better future.

Imagine yourself standing on a pathway. As you look around the left, right and above is brilliantly illuminated, and sounds are amazingly clear. As you check over your shoulder you notice the path behind is unclear. You hear a clock chime in the distance and take a step forward. You notice the slightest of noises, movements or shifts of light, and take pleasure even in the pure sound of silence, too. You can hear that same clock ticking now, and with each tick you can take a small step forward, effortlessly, along the path, and that illumination and awareness moves with you. At any fork in the path you can make decisions easily as you are truly involved in the moment, rather than looking over your shoulder at what might have been, or staring blindly into the future at what might happen. You enjoy being in the brilliantly illuminated, acute awareness of sound, hearing, feeling, taste and smell that is NOW.

For a complete experience, be more acutely aware of shapes and textures as well as sounds, colours and scents.

GOAL ACHIEVEMENT

A goal, in all areas of life, is vitally important in order to focus your attention and inner resources. A goal provides a sense of direction and ultimately the joy of achievement. Without it you might flounder, so keep saying to yourself …
- I direct my energies to achieve my goals.
- I enjoy directing my energies positively.
- I know where I am going and how I am getting there.
- Step by step I am moving in the right direction.
- I have the ability, I have the determination, I shall succeed.

Keep your eyes firmly fixed on your goal and you will achieve it.

Be aware of the different areas of your life: work, social, leisure activities, emotional and spiritual. Select one of these for this exercise … and be aware of what you want to happen in that area of your life, what you want to achieve … Make it realistic and clear in your mind. It may be useful to write it down and describe it fully before beginning this visualization.

While in the meditative state, imagine yourself having achieved that goal, imagine yourself there, in that situation. Surround yourself with all the things or people that indicate that you have achieved that goal. Be as specific as you can … be aware of all the senses … what are you seeing … hearing … touching or sensing … smelling … tasting. Be there … make it real … be specific … about colours … temperatures … lighting, to make it more and more real in your mind.

Now, from where you are at that moment of achieving that goal … look back … as if along a path, a pathway of time … to where you were … and notice the different stages of change … of movement towards achieving that goal … along the way … along that path … the different actions you have taken … the contacts you have made … and the people involved. Be aware of all the stages along the way … and as you return to the here and now … you remain in touch with the feelings that will make it all worthwhile … and you feel more and more determined to take one step at a time … make one change at a time … along that path to the successful achievement of your goal. And as you return from the meditative state so you are more determined to be successful in the achievement of your goal.

a

abdomen: yoga, 78–9
affirmations, meditation, 90–1
Alexander, Frederick Matthias, 14
Alexander technique, 13–29
alternate leg pulls, yoga, 76
arms:
    arm and back stretch, yoga, 81
    arm and chest stretch, yoga, 81
    arm circling, yoga, 68
    arm stretching, yoga, 69
attention, t'ai chi, 44

b

back:
    arm and back stretch, yoga, 81
    back push-up, yoga, 77
    back/shoulder stretch, yoga, 81
    posture clasp, yoga, 81
backache, yoga, 72–3
bend bow to shoot tiger, t'ai chi, 64
bending, Alexander technique, 22, 24, 25
bending twist, yoga, 73
biorhythms, 84
body/mind link, meditation, 92
brain, endorphins, 84
brush right knee and push, t'ai chi, 60

c

calf stretch, yoga, 80
carrying, Alexander technique, 26
cars, Alexander technique, 27
cat stretch, yoga, 69, 77, 80
Chi, 32
cobra, yoga, 72
colours, meditation, 85
computers, Alexander technique, 29
confidence, meditation and, 91
country house meditation, 89

d

deskwork, Alexander technique, 28
drinking, Alexander technique, 27
driving, Alexander technique, 27

e

eating, Alexander technique, 27
embrace tiger, return to mountain, t'ai chi, 51–2
endorphins, meditation, 84
energy, Chi, 32
eyes, Alexander technique, 18

f

fair lady weaves shuttle, t'ai chi, 61–2
forearm stretch, yoga, 81
full leg pulls, yoga, 76

g

goal achievement, meditation, 93
golden rooster stands on one leg, t'ai chi, 55–7
"Grasping the Sparrow's Tail", t'ai chi, 46
guided visit to a country house meditation, 89

h

handling, Alexander technique, 21
harmony, 10
haven meditation, 88
head, Alexander technique, 14
head to chest, yoga, 74

i

iron fan penetrates back, t'ai chi, 58–9

index

l

legs:
    leg over exercise, yoga, 78
    leg revivers, yoga, 76–7
lifting, Alexander technique, 26
lifting hands, t'ai chi, 47–8
lion posture, yoga, 74
living now, meditation, 93
loose twists, yoga, 69
lotus, yoga, 78
"lunge monkey", Alexander technique, 24
lying down, Alexander technique, 19
lying twists, yoga, 79

m

mantras, meditation, 85
meditation, 83–93
meridians, Chi, 32
mobile phones, Alexander technique, 29
"monkey", Alexander technique, 22

n

neck:
    Alexander technique, 14
    yoga, 74
neck twists, yoga, 80
needles at sea bottom, t'ai chi, 58
numbers game, meditation, 88

o

office work:
    Alexander technique, 28–9
    yoga, 80–1

p

personal development, meditation, 90–1
play guitar, brush left knee and push, t'ai chi, 49
posture:
    Alexander technique, 13–29
    yoga, 75
posture clasp, yoga, 81
punch under elbow, t'ai chi, 52

r

reaching, Alexander technique, 21
reading, Alexander technique, 28
relaxation:
    endorphins, 84
    meditation, 84
ride tiger, t'ai chi, 63–4
roll back, press and push, t'ai chi, 46, 52
roll twist, yoga, 79
Rossi, Ernest, 84

s

seated cat stretch, yoga, 80
self-esteem, meditation, 90
semi-supine position, Alexander technique, 19
semicircle rotation, yoga, 74
shake, yoga, 69
shoulders:
    Alexander technique, 14
    yoga, 68, 81
shrugging shoulders, yoga, 68
side bends, yoga, 79
side leg raise, yoga, 76
sideways bend, yoga, 69
sideways neck stretch, yoga, 74
single whip, t'ai chi, 47
sit up/lie down, yoga, 77, 79
sitting, Alexander technique, 20
slouch stress, yoga, 73
sound, meditation, 85
spine: Alexander technique, 14
squatting:
    Alexander technique, 24, 25
    yoga, 68
squatting single whip, step forward for seven stars, t'ai chi, 63
standing, Alexander technique, 20
step back to repulse the monkey, t'ai chi, 53
step forward, deflect downwards, intercept and punch, t'ai chi, 59

tiptoes, Alexander technique, 21
touch, meditation, 85
tree, yoga, 75
triangle, yoga, 73
20-minute rule, meditation, 84
twists, yoga, 69, 72–3, 79

u

ultradian rhythms, 84

v

visualization, meditation, 91

w

walking, t'ai chi, 43
ward off left, t'ai chi, 45
ward off left, ward off right, roll back, press and push, t'ai chi, 62
ward off right, roll back, press and push, t'ai chi, 60–1
ward off right, t'ai chi, 45
warm-up exercises:
    t'ai chi, 333-41
    yoga, 68–9
waving hands in clouds, t'ai chi, 54–5

well meditation, 89
"White Crane Spreads Wings and Push", t'ai chi, 48–9
withdraw and push, crossing hands t'ai chi, 50–1, 65
work, meditation and, 84
writing, Alexander technique, 28

y

yang-style short form, t'ai chi, 43–65
Yin and Yang, 32
yoga stretches, 67-81

step forward, deflect, intercept and punch, t'ai chi, 49–50
stress, 7
    meditation, 92
stretches, yoga, 67-81
"Strumming the Lute", t'ai chi, 49

t

t'ai chi, 31–65
Tan Tien, 32
telephones, Alexander technique, 29
tension, yoga, 72–4

Picture Acknowledgements

The majority of the pictures in this book were taken by Don Last and Dave Jordan. Additional photography by: Michelle Garrett, Simon Bottomley and Alistair Hughes.

The publishers would like to thank the following picture libraries for supplying pictures for use in this book: A-Z Botanical Collection Ltd: 86ML. Garden & Wildlife Matters: 93TR. Tony Stone Images: 84BL; 85BL; 87TR; 88TL, BR; 89TL, BR; 90BL; 91T; 93BL.